I know there are so many people with physical or mental health conditions. If this is you, in spirit, I sit with you. I acknowledge the struggle and the pain. I hope my story inspires you and gives you hope. Having been so unwell for so many years, I never imagined my body could heal and recover so well. Nor could I imagine my life would be so filled with love again.

dianneellis.com.au

Testimonies
'Dianne is a loving and compassionate angel and a true emissary of light in this world. Her vast knowledge gained through decades of research in overcoming her personal illnesses, combined with her unrelenting dedication in going to the depths of her body's wisdom, has fuelled an enormous fire within her to take her message to the world. In sharing her profound healing experiences, she brings joy, empowerment and enlightenment to those who hear her and has been a true inspiration to me and to so many who have attended my courses.'
Carol Roberts, Genome Healing Founder

'**MIRACLES** happen at Genome Healing courses ... and Di Ellis is living proof of that. Di's unwavering belief in Genome Healing's "heal, seal and protect" techniques has transformed her life of illness and suffering into a life full of energy and effervescence. What impresses me most about Di is not only that she has recreated her life, but also her expression of gratitude for the 'gift of healing' which she fully embraces. She truly is exemplary and an inspiring woman, full of joy and happiness and, above all, love, which she freely shares with anyone she encounters.'
Peter Murphy, Genome Healing Master

Copyright ©2019 by Dianne Ellis
Design & cover photo by Di Ellis
All rights reserved. No part of this book may be used or reproduced by any means, graphic, electronic, mechanical, including photocopying, recording, taping or by any information storage retrieval system without the written permission of the publisher except in the case of brief quotations embodied in critical articles and reviews.

Quantum Health

My Journey back from Lyme, Cancer and Chronic Illness

DIANNE ELLIS

Dedicated to ...

My beautiful first born, Jemma
My first to be born at home. First to have only home care and remedies when ill. First student in our homeschool. First to make me so proud of your caring, thoughtfulness and achieving, praised by the teachers when suddenly thrown into high school. Strongest in the home when I was ill. I always wanted to protect you from the hurts and loss that I experienced. It didn't quite work out that way. But you kept me here. You showed me giving up wasn't an option that you would accept. You looked after your sister when I couldn't. You pushed me to be strong when I was weak. You pushed me to keep going when I could see no light. I acknowledge how hard it's been for you. I know you think my 'clone', lol, is my favourite, but we would both be lost without you. I will always appreciate you more than you know. I will always love you more than you realise.

My Lily
Born on my birthday. Not quite my clone, lol. But close. You held me when I was broken. You lifted me when I was down. You carried everything when I couldn't. You understood when no one did. You stayed when others left. You believed in me even when we'd lost everything. You supported me in my darkest days. Few would realise the weight you have carried, but still a smile on your face, your softness so soothing and warm. All my love.

Our loved ones
Too many to mention but you know who you are. Friends, family, surrogate uncles, aunties and grandparents. As well as our sense of self, nothing is more important than our loved ones who walk by our sides. We are so blessed.

Health workers
To all of my holistic practitioners, healers, midwives, nurses, ground breaking doctors, researchers, mentors, teachers and truth seekers (some who have passed) who share their knowledge, wisdom and many secrets to life. Those who sat by me in the depths, nursed me and prayed for me. Thank you will never be enough to express my gratitude.

My soul sister Nikki
What a ride hey! Love you always.

Dad, my rock
I know you are always with me.

Jen, my mum
Not by blood, but spirit. It's hard to find words. Only feelings of being so loved, supported, wanted and appreciated. My heart is warm and full. A wholeness and contentedness like never before. What you give I return with all my heart. Thank you.

My love, Craig
You are everything I could ever ask for. You are my everything. Your kindness, caring and love melts my heart. You melt my heart.

Table of Contents

DISCLAIMER II
ACKNOWLEDGEMENTS II
INTRODUCTION II

PART 1
A MIRACULOUS JOURNEY OF LOVE, HEALING AND TRANSFORMATION 1
1 ITCHING TO BE FREE 2
2 A WALK BETWEEN WORLDS 6
3 MY ANGEL FROM HEAVEN 11
4 FLOATING ON A SEA OF UNCERTAINTY 20
5 THE EYE OF THE STORM 25
6 BORN TO BE 30
7 THE BREATH OF LIFE 35
8 THE BREATH OF HEAVEN 43
9 THE RIDE OF MY LIFE 46
10 PORTAL TO ANOTHER DIMENSION 57
11 DRAWN INTO A PRIMAL, DARK AND MAGICAL WORLD 61
12 SURRENDER 72
13 A PLACE OF DEEP LOVE AND CONNECTION 76
14 SHARK ATTACK 80
15 ALLOWED TO LOVE 83
16 THE BEAUTY BENEATH LIFE AND DEATH 91
17 SOME ANSWERS AT LAST 102
18 WISE OLD MEN 108
19 A WORLD BETWEEN WORLDS 113
20 LUCKY ESCAPE 123
21 SINISTER SWEETNESS 127
22 POSITIVE RESULTS 134
23 REFLECTIONS 142
24 BACK TO WHERE IT ALL BEGAN 147

25 HEALING AT WARP SPEED 152
26 WHEN WORLDS COLLIDE 165

PART 2
SUMMARY OF MY HEALING PROTOCOL **183**
WHAT I WISH I KNEW THEN 184
HIDDEN CAUSES OF CHRONIC ILLNESS.. 184
HIDDEN CAUSES OF ANXIETY AND DEPRESSION 185
KISS – KEEP IT SIMPLE SWEETHEART! 186
BASIC PROTOCOL … STEP BY STEP **187**
THE HEALING JOURNEY 192
EXTENSIVE PROTOCOL … RECOVERY OF OPTIMUM HEALTH.............**204**
   1 DETOX 205
   2 STRESS RELEASE AND POSITIVE INTENTION 213
   3 DIET/GUT HEALTH 214
   4 ALKALIZE YOUR BODY 218
   5 ACTIVATE YOUR BODY'S OWN SELF-HEALING MECHANISMS..................... 220
   6 ELIMINATE PATHOGENS … PARASITES, VIRUSES AND BACTERIA, MOULD AND CANDIDA.. 226
   7 BALANCE BIOCHEMISTRY... 234
   8 REALIGN YOUR BODY 235
   9 EXERCISE 236
   10 ENERGY HEALING... 237
   11 EMOTIONAL HEALING … RELEASE TRAUMAS AND THE EMOTIONAL CONNECTION TO PHYSICAL ILLNESS.. 246
   12 SOUL HEALING 252
   VENTURING OUT … WITH YOUR INNER SELF 260
   MY ONGOING HEALTH RECOVERY PROTOCOL 264

Disclaimer

All material in this book is purely for informational purposes. The opinions and methods outlined are not intended to provide direct treatment of physical, mental, or emotional illnesses and diseases. It is not intended to diagnose, treat, cure or prevent any disease by direct means, beyond the help of qualified fully certified practitioners.

Acknowledgements

I would like to acknowledge the work of all holistic practitioners, researchers, scientists and engineers whose heart-felt work contributes to the health and wellbeing of humanity every day. While I share a lot of information in this book, it's only a small piece of the vast amount of information, experience and knowledge that is available.

Introduction

I invite you to join me on a journey. A journey of healing through time and space to some of the deepest, darkest mystical places of the soul. I offer this experience so you can become part of this journey, to feel it, and gain an understanding of what might be occurring in yourself or someone close. Are your feelings, your illness, or your circumstances calling you to venture on your own inner journey? To find a deeper love and understanding of yourself, your loved ones, or your life.

When I first became unwell thirty years ago I never imagined the journey ahead. There have been many times when I didn't know if I would live or die. Many times that I just didn't have the strength to keep trying. After a lifetime of chronic ill-health I gave up on reclaiming my previously unbridled energy. I learnt to put up with and find peace in feeling unwell. But after receiving a number of tick bites, the excruciating symptoms which ensued were unbearable. I bounced from doctor to naturopath, hospital to homeopath and every other practitioner I could find. Nothing stopped my descent into a serious life-threatening condition. I had to find something, anything to escape this hell. Would I ever find my way back? I thought it impossible to be active and healthy again.

I now know the deep trauma and grief I have experienced in my life is deeply interwoven with my chronic illnesses. When we find the way to unlock and release trauma from our body and remove the underlying causes of ill-health, our body has an amazing self-healing ability. Likewise, when we delicately untangle and reframe the negative thought patterns and beliefs which underlie our illness, joy, love and happiness will often spontaneously and unexpectedly fill our lives.

Herein I pass on the wisdom I've acquired through my own trials and tribulations, combined with the wisdom and teachings that have been passed on to me by incredible healers, shamans, and every day simple folk. When I was gravely ill one of my practitioners held my hands every day, praying that I would recover, reassuring me that I would get through this and go on to help others going through similar circumstances. So that's just what I'm doing now. I share with you the results of years of searching and researching conventional and unconventional medical practices, and everything in between. Experimenting, trial and error with many different treatments, remedies, potions and lotions until I discovered a few simple home remedies and medical breakthroughs to activate our body's own self-healing mechanisms quickly and effectively. Here I also share my experiences of adoption, death, separation and deep grief. The beauty and healing power of nature and the ocean. I also detail the methods which enabled me to come to peace with some of the most traumatic events and relationships in my life, and how I came to the realisation that each one of them actually represented a part of myself, a very deep subconscious part of me that had given up on life due to the pain I had experienced. I hope to give you, the reader, a sense of the journey forward amid the day-to-day experiences we still have to deal with on our wider healing quest and life in general.

For those of you who are seriously unwell and desperately in need of information quickly, I have included a summary of the treatments, methods and remedies that have not only been most beneficial for my health recovery but no doubt saved my life, at the end of this book. These are provided as a guide to help you find the appropriate professional advice, and enough information to enable you to ask more informed questions in your quest for health.

Di Ellis

Part 1

A Miraculous Journey of Love, Healing and Transformation

1 Itching to be Free

Walking along a beautiful beach the incoming tide urges me higher up the sand. The waves suddenly seem to be getting bigger pushing me further up the beach. I scramble over the rocks at the bottom of the cliff searching for higher ground. The waves are relentless. Rising even more, they come closer and closer. I feel panic rushing through my body as I ascend the cliff face with foamy water reaching for my feet. Quickly, I climb as high as I can. Sand and stones fall away under my fingers. I gasp for breath. Sheer cliff above, I cannot go higher. I look around. Another wave is coming, even bigger than the last. In fright I awake.
Twenty years later, we've just moved north to a coastal town. As I walk along the beach I marvel at the serene beauty. The sandstone cliffs patterned with colors of chocolate, caramel and vanilla swirl. Small waterfalls dripping down from the pandanas roots hanging precariously over the cliff. My daughters, Jemma and Lily, are playing at the water's edge. I look around and I'm suddenly shocked by what I see. This is my dreamscape. The location of a recurring dream I had as a child. The cove, the rocks, the cliff. I feel the adrenalin sweep over my body as it has done in my dreams many times. Automatically, I examine how big the waves are. I check for an escape route. Taking a deep breath I give myself a shake.
"Don't be silly," I tell myself. "This is fine. That was a dream, it's not real."
I feel very strange for a while. I know I have never been here before, but I cannot explain this bizarre experience.
How I crave for a simple quiet life. Little do I realise all the feelings I experienced within my dream; the fear, the panic, not knowing if I will survive, will become a reality. It's New Year's Eve 1999. Moving back north away from the cold just a few days ago it's so good to feel warm, safe and peaceful. After living in the bush for so long, it feels strange to be around so many people. I can't help but look at each person I walk past and nod at them in acknowledgment. I'm getting some strange reactions. I have forgotten this beautiful seaside town with its holidaymakers is not the same as our small country township, which was home for a bit over three years.
Tomorrow will be the new millennium. I'm not excited. I'm weary and with two young girls, who are only one and three years old. So it's an early night for us. To my dismay, people everywhere are letting off fire crackers. I jump each time I hear one.

Di Ellis

I tell myself over and over, "It's fine; it's just a fire cracker."
But still it feels like a shock wave jolting through my body. It sounds so much like a gun shot. I'm relieved as we move into the New Year and everything calms down. Living in such a beautiful area, it's easy to feel at home quickly. Over the following years I do as much as I can to make my life as simple and quiet as possible, so much so that the spark I used to have within has died. So has my marriage.

I've been on my own with the girls for a couple of years now. Moving back into our home, surrounded by beautiful countryside not far from the beach, this truly is paradise. I get into the garden clearing weeds, creating new vegetable plots, herb spirals and ponds for the frogs. I begin to convert the garage into a therapy room for my breathwork practice. We buy day old chicks, which the girls nurture and carry around all day. Hanging high on the back of our house is a nesting box for the local parrots, who are working hard preparing their nest as we head into spring. Vines and weeds have woven their way through the clothesline, which has been lying on the ground. It's a big job untangling it all. Eventually I'm able to lift it up and prop it against a big old tree stump, which I keep as an interesting feature in the yard. Later in the afternoon, with great satisfaction, I tackle the last clump of weeds with the mower. That afternoon I find three ticks burrowing into my ear. I pull them out and have a shower to wash away any others. With pleasure and surprise I watch yet another few disappear down the plughole. I'm infested with the horrible little creatures! That evening I pull the eighth and final tick from the top of my head.

Immediately I feel a wave of heat rush through my body, turning my skin bright red, my eyes bloodshot. My heart is thumping desperately. It feels like it's going to jump through my chest. My head spins. I lie down quickly to avoid passing out. I try to act calm so not to scare the girls. A friend drops in. I'm relieved to have him sit with me. At my request the girls go and get a neighbour who is a pharmacist. I figure he might have some advice and hopefully some antihistamines, but he is reluctant to give me anything and feels I should go to the doctor. For many years now I've taken full responsibility for my own health and prefer not to see a doctor unless absolutely essential so I just wait to see how things go. Gradually I start to feel a little better, thank my friends for their care and tell them I will be okay.

All night I'm jolted awake with muscle twitches and spasms. I'm feverish and dripping in sweat. The next day I ring my friend Averil who is a nurse. She's very knowledgeable about mainstream medicine and many different forms of natural therapies in part due to her journey of recovery from multiple sclerosis. She warns me of something called Lyme disease, says it's not worth mucking around with and recommends I see a doctor. Although I've not had antibiotics for many years I take what is prescribed. I'm also given anti-histamines in case of future tick bites. By the next evening I'm relieved to be almost back to normal.

The girls and I love our time at the beach walking, swimming and surfing. I don't surf a lot though. Not the way I used to. For many years a persistent underlying fatigue has held me back from doing many things. It's been very disheartening watching the other surfers while I have little energy to be out there. I've battled with my health all my life. As a child I had bad asthma, at times very severe. I was still extremely active though. I guess at times hyperactive. A real tomboy. In my late teens I had a bad flu, which I later discovered was Ross River Fever, from which I never fully recovered. Digestive disorders and chronic fatigue soon set in. For a couple of years I took whatever treatment the doctors suggested; medication, injections, operations, tablets, sprays and vaccinations. My condition only worsened. Nothing gave me relief. I sought natural therapies, changed to a healthier diet and avoided toxins as much as possible. Although my health improved somewhat I never regained my previous vitality. After many years of fluctuations in my health, I gave up trying to work out what was wrong. I recovered enough energy to lead a fairly active life so all that was left was to accept the way things were, persist and push on.

The surfing adventures of my younger days are becoming a distant memory, driving up and down the coast with my good friend Nikki in her bright yellow Torana with a big peace sign painted on the bonnet, looking for the best waves.

One day with a car full of girls, as usual the petrol gauge is sitting precariously below empty. We are only around the corner from home but inevitably we don't make it that far.

"Oh no, not again," we all chorus.

"You lot'll have to push," says Nikki laughing.

Kim, Leanne and I hop out and start pushing while Nik steers. Mel grabs the guitar and climbs on the roof. Sitting cross-legged she happily strums away, singing a song in which we all join in.

"Woohoo," some muscly surfie guys with sun bleached hair howl and toot as they drive past.

With excitement we cheer and return the gesture. A couple sitting on their front veranda giggle at the sight in front of them.

Di Ellis

"Hi," we call, waving happily.
Down the road, an older man is walking along the footpath.
"Do you want to help us push?" I ask.
"I guess so, why not?"
"You have to sing though."
To our amusement, he joins in with our song as we all push the car home. Events like this become the normal way to spend our weekends full of mischief and fun.
It's around 10 pm and the nightlife in Surfers Paradise is just beginning to awaken. There's the usual buzz of electricity in the air and the streets are alive with people as Nikki and I make our way to meet friends at a local bar. Along the way, to our delight, we're entertained by a busker who's happy to play some of our favourite songs as we twirl and dance on the footpath. Slowly a larger crowd gathers, people join in our dance and to the busker's delight, his hat quickly fills. Almost an hour since creating our own dance floor, we figure it's time to make our way to the next one.
"Oh, you're not going are you?" says the busker.
"Thanks for the great music," we say giving him a hug goodbye. At the next venue we are the first on the dance floor which quickly fills with party goers and free drinks are provided for our efforts.
After having children that wild, free, forever-young part of myself shut down. I focused on being a good mother and giving my girls the best I could. I guess I thought I was just being a good responsible mother, which of course I was, but I had no clue of the incredible lifeforce within me that I was also closing down. A lifeforce which provides vibrancy, health and sustenance. I thought those wild reckless days must have been, in some regard, a product of my misplaced childhood. Little did I realise they were in fact a very valuable expression of a part of myself. Never did I think that part of me was intrinsically connected to my deepest fears, waiting to present themselves in so many terrifying ways. Nor could I have imagined that deep within that terror was the key to my health, and the deepest wisdom and love I have ever known.

2 A Walk Between Worlds

Life now with the girls is home-schooling, crafts, painting, and science experiments. Watching rosellas while studying our bird book, or outings with the home-school group. This wonderful group of people have organised a day for the kids to experience medieval life. Arriving at our friend's property it really does look as though we've gone back in time. Boys run attacking each other with swords, while the girls admire each other's dresses, jumping in on the fighting when they see an opportunity. I add my dish to the amazing banquet on the table. After a wonderful day of feasting and medieval activities we thank our hosts and make our way home.

It's six months since my bad reaction to the tick bites. Once again I find myself removing ticks, which have decided I make a pretty nice meal. I've been over the road to see my neighbour, ninety four year-old Mrs Honeyman still living at home. Inevitably she is down in the garden planting seedlings or picking fruit. As I walk between two bushes it crosses my mind about ticks, but it's a fairly clear area near the road so I assume it's fine.

Later in the afternoon I start to itch. This time the ticks are tiny. Smaller than a pin head. I'm much more careful than last time. I realise that pulling them out you can actually squeeze the venom into yourself. So far I've had very little reaction, though I fear one. So I drop in to see my homeopath Ilma who gives me a remedy in case I need it. Returning home I notice my body becoming hot and my heart beginning to race. Immediately I take the remedy, which works incredibly well. I have a shower to wash away any other ticks and I'm relieved to have very few symptoms as I doze off to sleep.

Sudden muscle twitches jolt me from my relaxed sleep. My pyjamas are dripping with sweat. My heart is racing. Shivering and shaking I quickly turn on the light to search for more ticks. Sure enough I find about twenty. I cover myself in eucalyptus oil and take antihistamines. To my dismay, they do nothing. I take more homeopathic remedy, which eases things somewhat and in the morning I go to the doctor for another course of antibiotics.

For the next week my symptoms persist. The homeopathic remedy gives me temporary relief but the sweats, shivering, shaking and muscle twitches keep returning. Day and night I'm exhausted from lack of sleep.

Di Ellis

Beating erratically my heart leads me to believe that something is quite wrong. Time to take myself to hospital.
The doctor, diagnoses anxiety, offering me Valium. A sudden image overwhelms my mind, body and all of my senses. In my mind's eye I see my step mother standing at the entrance to a hospital. A psychiatric hospital. She's been here for two weeks receiving shock treatment. She's in a white robe as all the patients are, walking around like zombies. I'm in the car with Dad and my sister and we're just leaving.
"Go and see if your mother is all right," Dad says, watching her leaning sleepily against the doorframe.
I don't want to go back there. Not near her, those people, or that place.
"She's fine," I say crossly, and we drive away.
I refuse to take the Valium.
"The ticks have set your anxiety off," insists the doctor, trying to convince me otherwise.
I have suffered from plenty of anxiety over the years, so it's not new to me. Yet I know there is something else causing these awful physical symptoms. Despite this current nightmare, there is no way in the world I will touch Valium.
Over the following weeks my condition doesn't improve. Now I really am becoming very scared and anxious. I take myself for short walks along my favourite beach. Here I am living my dream, that feels more like a nightmare. I look around at the rocks, the cliff and the beach. I'm not scared of the waves in the ocean, but I'm terrified of these sensations rippling through my body. All day, all night, I'm feverish with muscle twitches and heart palpitations. I push myself to accept an invitation to lunch. Maybe getting out with some friends will make me feel better.
Unfortunately I don't feel well enough to enjoy my meal, or being out with the girls. One of my friends tells me about a book she has that explains the detrimental effects of eating grains and drops it over the next day. It's interesting reading and seems to correlate with what's happening with my health, so I cut all grains out of my diet. It's amazing. I don't know why but suddenly my health is back to normal. I'm feeling better than I have in a very long time. How blissful it is to have a restful night's sleep, to return to some normal activities including riding my horses.
I've been passionate about surfing for a long time, but I've also had a deep love for horses since I was young. As I will learn, holding onto what brings joy and love to your life is so important when finding your way through chronic illness. My first horse Cobba was heading towards thirty years old

when he passed. He was five when my parents bought him for me and I was thirteen. While many of the girls were chasing boys I just wanted to get home from school to be with my faithful companion. It wasn't a rare thing for me to saddle him up and disappear for the day. During my last visit with him he went and lay down under a tree. Sitting beside him I told him how much I loved him and thanked him for being there for me for so many years.

I've rescued many horses over the years. I'm not sure if I was saving them or they were saving me. Each time I visit them now I notice how many ticks are crawling up their necks or burrowing into their skin. Occasionally I find one crawling on me. Every time I touch the horses or walk to them through the long grass I'm wary and fearful. I hate being this way. But at least I'm feeling pretty good so I try not to let my fear hold me back. Memories of riding weekends away are becoming another distant memory.

My old riding mate Lennie, his wife Barb and daughter Dana recently came to visit. We were looking through old photos reminiscing about all our adventures and good friends including Steve and Jacqui.

"Have you seen Steve lately?" I ask.

"I've seen him a couple of times but not for a while. He doesn't drive buses anymore so I don't see him at work. Wow, what have we got here?"

Jemma, Lily and Dana come running out all dressed up as hula girls, singing, dancing and laughing. Lennie picks up my sarong. Wrapping it around his waist as a skirt he runs around the house chasing the girls and dancing the hula with them.

"Alright, come on kids, let's go into town," he says.

"You get that skirt off first," Barb insists.

"I think he looks better like that Barb."

She shakes her head at him.

"I need to go and do a few jobs first, but I'll meet you in there," I say.

"What, are you running off to see a secret bloke?" teases Lennie.

"For me to know and you not to find out," I laugh.

Having finished my errands, I park the car in town and see the others walking along the footpath towards me. When I hop out of the car, I look over at Lennie who's looking at me in a very strange way. He then looks in confusion at someone standing just in front of me, then back at me, and back to the other person again. I look in curiosity at the man he is staring at, and then back to Lennie.

"Steve," he yells.

"Steve?" I say, as I approach the man.

Di Ellis

To our shock and amazement our dear friend who we have just been reminiscing about is standing in front of us, on holiday a couple of hours from home. He is just as shocked and surprised as we are. We all stand in the street laughing, jumping and hugging each other before making out way back home to once again go through all the old photos together.
"There's you on that goldy coloured horse of yours Steve, galloping on the beach. What was his name?'
"Norman," Steve replies with a huge smile on his face seeing the photo.
Having crossed the Noosa River on the ferry, we drive into the camping ground, unload the horses and put them in the stables. After lunch and unloading our gear at the bunkhouse everyone is keen for a ride. We saddle up the horses and find the path that leads to the beach. Riding for a couple of kilometres along a narrow dirt track through the coastal scrub, we all anticipate our arrival at the beach.
"There it is!" I exclaim seeing the water through the trees. The horses hooves sink into the sand as we walk towards the water. They are very wary of the waves.
"Come on Cob. It won't hurt you," I squeeze his belly with my heels.
He walks side to side, avoiding going forward. The water recedes and I coax him on. A wave washes towards us and I'm happy to stay on when he jumps away suddenly.
"It's alright boy," I rub his neck and push him forward.
All the horses are shying backwards and forwards as their riders encourage them closer. We walk along the beach at the water's edge, but walking doesn't last long. The horses are stirred up. Shaking their heads, they try to gain freedom from the bridles that are restricting them. They are just as excited as their riders who are ready to go. Cobba, eager to gallop, begins to jump around knocking into Steve's horse beside us. I feel the pressure on my leg, squashed between the two horses. I feel their energy, their power, the warmth of their bodies. I love this.
We all break into a trot, which quickly speeds up to a canter. Steve stands up in the saddle. Outstretching his arm, he points forward yelling, "Charge!" as we all burst into a full gallop.
"Yeeehaaaaa!"
Leaning forward, holding on tight, manes flying in the air, I look around at everyone as we race each other along the beach. Filled with exhilaration, we're all silent. Just the sound of the horse's hooves pounding on the firm sand, the flaring of their nostrils as they breath, the crash of waves nearby. A faster horse moves ahead leaving those of us in its path pelted with sand. I quickly pull Cobba to the side. Wiping sand off

my face I'm relieved to be able to see again. Soon the horses begin to tire and gradually slow down. We enjoy our ride in awe. Eventually the horses become more confident in the water. Cantering through the shallow waves majestically, they lift their legs high, spray reaching up into the air, showering us all.
Remember the moonlight rides, cantering down the middle of the road, sparks from the horses shoes flying.
"They were wild days weren't they?" says Steve.
"And weren't they fun," agrees Lennie.
Later as he leaves to head home, he adds, "You've got to eat up girl. You're fading away."
"Yeah, I know,' I agree, 'I just can't put weight on. But I'm trying."

3 My Angel From Heaven

I miss having family nearby, but we have a great community. As the weeks go by my health is slowly deteriorating. Despite my efforts to avoid them, I keep getting more tick bites. Even just walking to the car in the driveway I brush past a few sprigs of grass and soon notice a tick on my leg. I can't believe it. I wonder why they like me so much, while no one else seems to be getting so many. The homeopathic remedy is effective at reducing my reactions but not eliminating them. I find myself visiting my horses less frequently. Everywhere I go I avoid any long grass. I start to notice how much more weight I'm losing. This is not good as I'm already too thin. I eat a huge amount of food but my weight is still dropping. I'm reacting to more and more foods, needing to eliminate more from my diet.

I see a naturopath who uses kinesiology, muscle testing for any weakness I may have due to any food allergies or emotional issues. Kinesiology is a form of muscle testing to identify imbalances in the body's structural, chemical, mental, emotional or other energy. It is an effective way of letting our body do the talking, bypassing all the misinformation and theoretical possibilities we often have swirling around in our head when we feel unwell. I like kinesiology as it allows me and all my worries to take a back seat, and let my body do the talking. I'm always amazed at how accurately it pinpoints how I really am, as opposed to how I think I am at any one time.

My naturopath is working on my food allergies. She gives me a vial of food or a substance to hold while she presses down on my out held arm. If my arm is weak it shows my body is weakened by that substance. If my arm holds firm it shows the substance is not causing me any problem. Her methodical testing confirms that I'm sensitive to a number of things such as milk and house dust mites. I'm given some supplements, which seem helpful, but again the benefits are only temporary. Realising I really need more help I see a specialist GP who also practises complementary medicine. To my delight he is very receptive to my naturopath's findings, but also focused on running a series of extensive tests to try and find out what else might be going on. Most of the results are quite good even giving me a body age of twenty-nine. At thirty-nine years of age I'm pretty chuffed about that but I know I'm certainly supposed to be feeling better than this.

The tests show that my body is suffering the signs of malabsorption. This I'm advised is the result of parasites and an inflamed bowel. I'm given

black seed capsules to kill parasites but my symptoms are aggravated so badly that I don't persist. Thorough testing also shows a thyroid imbalance with low levels of T3, a thyroid hormone called triiodothyronine. It seems many doctors only test for TSH and sometimes T4, therefore this problem often goes undetected. Thyroid Stimulating Hormone known as TSH, is a hormone produced and released into the bloodstream by the pituitary gland which tells the thyroid gland how much T4 and T3 to produce. T4 is another thyroid hormone called thyroxine. Medication doesn't help and once again makes me feel worse. I later discover many people with hypothyroidism and Hashimoto's have low levels of T3 and the cause of the problem is usually either damage to the thyroid gland caused by the immune system or a problem converting T4 to T3. I mention to the doctor that I often have a sensation just below my ribs like a stitch. Sometimes I can feel a lump there. Gently he presses on my abdomen.
"Yes, I can feel something there. I think you'd better have an ultrasound."
I feel my abdomen fill with dread, but to my relief the tests come back clear. I continue to look for answers and seek more natural therapies, but nothing slows my downhill slide.
My meditation class holds a workshop creating mandalas, sacred patterns including circles and geometric shapes. My girls join us. Using coloured pens, pencils, crayons, pieces of paper, glitter and decorations, flowers, bark, rocks and glue in the centre of the table we create our individual designs. A kaleidoscope of colors and textures come to life in circular reflected patterns. Numerous ancient religions used mandalas to depict the cosmos and the pure sacred realm of spiritual existence. The mandala, meaning circle, exists in every aspect of life from a snail's shell, the rings of a tree, a snowflake, our own cells, the sun, the moon and our entire galaxy. Also contained within these shapes is the Fibonacci sequence, a mathematical equation found throughout nature.
Soothing music plays as I look around at everyone, at my beautiful girls, drawn into a deep meditative state, into the centre of their own little world on the paper as their creation comes to life. The end results are stunning pieces of work, some earthy and textured, while others are soft with flowing psychedelic colours. With surprising depth we all share the thoughts and feelings which our creations brought forward. Somehow, during these simple creative processes we are able to connect with and provide an avenue of expression for our subconscious mind. The place where so many feelings and emotions can remain hidden from our

awareness. I am learning what a valuable healing tool the creative arts can be.

I begin painting to distract me from everything. I've never been much of a painter but I learnt a few tips from my girls' teacher. As my health deteriorates so do my thoughts, emotions and feelings, connecting me once again with past traumas. I know we all experience traumas, sometimes burying them, other times able to deal with them well. I thought mine were all in the past, but now my sensitive state of health has brought them to the fore. I find myself pouring all of these emotions into my painting. I feel myself caught in a whirlwind of torment; my adopted mother's hospital bed where she was quarantined, watching her as a three year old in her last days on earth, my dream of the waves and the cliffs and, as I will soon discover, my future home, all reveal themselves in the painting in front of me. I don't know how, but in some way through this painting I'm connecting to a deep primal, but also higher part of myself.

Months pass and each day I struggle with my health. Despite eating huge amounts of vegetables and protein I'm severely underweight and becoming very weak. Each time I try to eat more carbohydrates, my reactions are so bad I just can't do it. I feel humiliated when people think I'm just not eating properly, or that I'm simply anxious. I know there is something wrong and I'm desperately trying to find out what it is. The more my health declines the more fearful I become. I'm bewildered at my lack of answers. I need to be well, if not for myself, for my girls. As usual I put on a positive face but inside I'm terrified. I have always been determined I would never leave my girls to face the kind of things I had to face in my childhood.

Finally one late October evening feeling like I'm going to pass out I call a friend and ask her to take me to the hospital where I spend a week. My health continues to decline. Most of my blood tests are within the normal range. There are a few things not quite right but nothing important. The doctors certainly aren't explaining why I feel like I'm going to die. Now I'm reacting to every single thing I eat. My chest is lighting up with a burning sensation, pain through my whole body. All of my muscles are cramping and my heart racing madly. I'm exhausted just resting. Night after night I can't sleep. This is a living hell.

I can eat very few things on the hospital menu so I'm grateful when my friend Danni brings in fresh food each day. Other friends look after the girls and bring them to visit regularly. I try to be cheerful, but I'm so fearful of leaving them. I know what it feels like to lose your mother.

More than anything I want to be there for them, to watch and support them as they grow. But I don't know how that can happen. I'm so sick and only becoming sicker. I think about the times I've been angry with them and I worry that if I die they might think they were not good enough so I write them a note telling them how much I love them and how wonderful they are. I hide it under the bed just in case I don't wake up.

White sheets, sterile hospital bed, silver metal, machines beeping. I cannot stand hospitals. Finding nothing in particular wrong with me, the doctors recommend anti-depressants. Again I refuse them. There is no way I'm going to take them. I want to know what is actually wrong with me. My birth mother who has been at a family function a few hours drive away comes to visit. It's comforting to see her, but also a little strained. We got on well when we first met when I was twenty-one years old but we've had our ups and downs since then.

I know I've had a lot of grief and trauma in my life, so I go over and over in my mind whether this could possibly be the cause of these awful symptoms. I have done so much therapy, so much deep healing, I just can't see how this sickness could be only anxiety. By the end of the week with no answers many of the doctors and nurses tell me these are symptoms of anxiety. Despite being certain there is something else wrong I give in. Maybe the traumas and grief from my past *have* somehow built up to cause these horrendous physical symptoms in my body. I accept Xanax. I'm also given beta blockers to slow down my rapid heartbeat although it doesn't seem to help.

Now I'm really starting to feel like I'm losing my mind. I've always been very strong in who I am and how I want my life to be. I have so much in life to look forward to. But now I can't think clearly and I don't like it one little bit. Everything becomes confused. Yet I'm too scared to stop taking the medication just in case it's going to work. With nothing else the hospital can do for me, I'm sent home. I'm despairing and disappointed. How can they possibly not find anything I wonder? I have never felt such a helpless sense of desperation. Thank God our dear fellow home-schooling friends Deb and Travis from up the coast come with their kids for a week to help out. I feel pathetic. I can't look after myself let alone my children. I have no idea how I'm going to overcome this. All I can do is struggle to survive each day. I don't realise it at the time, but it's going to take a long and agonising four years to discover that not only is my physical condition a part of Lyme disease, but so too are many of the severe symptoms of anxiety.

Later in the week my birth sister and her husband come to visit. Gratefully I accept their offer for my girls and I to stay with them for a while. Arriving in their home town I see the local doctor. It's the usual blood tests with the usual results. Everything looks fairly normal or at least within acceptable range. Yet my condition is still declining and I have very little health left to lose. My whole system is on fire. Any loud noises feel like an electric shock through my body. The same happens when I am touched. Having always been so affectionate with my girls, this agony when they hug me is unimaginable. Like an electric shock is going through me. I try to hide this hell from them, and do my best to give them the little love I can. My weight is critically low and dropping despite adding more carbohydrates to my diet. My sister who has been such an amazing support comes up with a plan to monitor what I'm eating.

The results baffle the doctor. Though I'm eating good meals my weight continues to drop. I realise they might have thought I was anorexic and possibly not eating much while in fact I've probably been eating more than many people do in my desperate bid to put on weight. All day, all night, my symptoms are tortuous. It's much worse within half an hour of eating. Burning feelings fill my chest. Tingling and muscle cramps throughout my body. Sweats. Muscle twitches and my heart racing and thumping as if it wants to jump through my chest. Night after night I can't sleep. I know I need something but I don't know what. This is horrific. With these drugs everything is like a bad dream. My mind is spinning. I cannot focus my attention or pull my thoughts together. Everything is a daze, my feelings a blur. One thing I do know … I am dying.

I need to do something, anything. One last hope, my mother makes an appointment with her naturopath. Petra lives about four hours away and my appointment is in a few days. I wonder if I will last that long. I am desperate. I speak to her on the phone and explain how I'm feeling.

"You need to come straight away. I want to see you this afternoon," she tells me.

My sister and her husband are such a pillar of strength. They drive me to see Petra, while my mother makes plans for me to stay with her friends Greg and Pam, who live nearby. I hate leaving my girls, unsure what might happen. I am so scared. I don't want them to lose their mother.

Petra is my angel from heaven. She studies my blood tests and finds many things she isn't happy with. "That's way too high," she says pointing to my liver enzyme levels. "One more point and it would be classified as high. At your age it should be much lower, in the middle somewhere. We need to get your electrolytes balanced too. Your sodium is too low."

I don't really know what she's talking about but at least something is happening. I later learn that congestion of the liver can have a huge influence on virtually every area of our health. And the balance of the electrolytes is vital for normal cell and organ function. I explain that every time I try to take any of the medication I've been given I feel worse.

"Your liver's really not handling it," Petra explains.

I share my fears wondering whether I will make it.

Taking my hands in hers she says, "Look at me Dianne. You are going to get through this. And then you will be able to help other people going through similar things."

Petra spends a very long time using muscle testing, methodically checking all of my organs, my response to any pathogens, viruses, parasites or bacteria that may be in my system, and which herbs, oils or supplements will be the most beneficial. Each time she places a remedy on my stomach she tests the strength in my arms and legs, some remedies making my body weak while others make me stronger. She finds a number of supplements my body seems to respond well to.

"Ok, now we just have to see if they go well together," she explains as she puts them all on my stomach and lifts my arm to see what my body tells her through its muscle response.

"Resist," she instructs many times until she isolates four supplements. It's quite exhausting but it gives me much more hope than I've had in a long time.

"Is that all?" I ask amazed.

She nods assuring me it's all my body is wanting right now. To finish my treatment Petra gives me a beautiful aromatherapy massage. "These oils are very powerful,' she tells. 'Good for killing parasites and bacteria, boosting the immune system and calming the nerves."

Somewhere beneath these awful sensations in my body, for a few moments I feel a sense of calm. Petra gives me Juniper berry tea to flush out my kidneys. I'm to add it to a cup of boiled water half an hour before each meal. She explains we have to cleanse the kidneys first so they can handle what is released when the liver is cleansed.

"Here's a mixture of Bach flower remedies, that will help your emotions. And here's some essential Lavender oil and Ylang Ylang to calm your nerves. And this is good for fighting parasites," Petra says giving me a sprig of tarragon from her garden."

I am also given MSM (methylsulfonylmethane), an organic sulphur compound used to help treat many illnesses and diseases, reduce pain and inflammation, and improve immune function. MSM provides biologically active sulphur, which is the fourth most plentiful mineral in the body and needed for many different critical bodily functions every single day.

Petra tells me that my blood type is A+ and that I should follow the diet suitable for that blood group, including chicken and turkey, most seafood and a selected variety of beans, nuts, fats, vegetables and fruit. I don't remember my blood type and I'm not sure how accurate she is, plus I really don't like legumes all that much, but subsequent tests prove that she is correct. Following my appointment Petra gives me a lift back to where I'm staying. I feel very lucky and secure to be just down the road from her. For now I'm to see her daily.

I don't look forward to the evenings. I miss the luxurious deep sleep that has blessed me my whole life. Until recently I've never understood how some people can't sleep properly. Feeling so awful all the time is bad enough but to have to put up with it all night when I should be soundly asleep is not at all enjoyable. I do my best to sleep but toss and turn most of the night. I awake in the early hours and my head is spinning. I truly feel like I have lost my mind. In confusion I don't know whether to call Petra, my mother or a psychiatric ward. I sit up and remind myself where I am. I tell myself over and over that everything is okay.

If only I could see ahead in time when I learn these are common Lyme disease symptoms. As usual I watch the windows hour after hour waiting to see the dark sky become light. After drifting in and out of sleep I'm relieved to finally see the changing colour in the sky and light streaming through the windows. I'm particularly relieved to have a reasonably clear mind. I used to love getting up early in the morning walking along the beach as the sun rose above the horizon but lying here for hours waiting for day to break, night after night, is utterly miserable. I never understood why some people with illness couldn't try to be a little happier, but I see now that chronic and serious illness can strip away all joy leaving just sadness, feeling vulnerable and frightened for the future.

"Normally we'd spend longer on your kidneys, but we have to get that liver cleaned out," says Petra the next day. Following my second appointment, with careful and thorough muscle testing, I'm given another herbal tea this time for my liver. I take it that day and again in the evening. The next morning on waking I feel like I have a football under my ribs. My liver is very swollen. It feels like I have a stitch, but it doesn't really hurt. I'm a little fearful and wonder what is going on but mostly I'm so glad that *something* is happening. Even a change like this is hope that

I might have some sort of improvement. Later in the day I need to go to the toilet and I know the liver cleanse is working. This is my turning point. I see Petra nearly every day for a week, then every couple of days the next week. My reactions after eating are still severe and I'm extremely unwell. Despite being filled with fear and dread each day I can feel my health is no longer declining. I even begin to put on weight. I had been very wary of using the oils, but Petra talks me into having another go.
"You need them to help your body settle!" she affirms.
Reluctantly I rub the Ylang Ylang on my ears. Almost immediately a wave of relief sweeps over my body. I don't know what it's doing, but it feels good. Thereafter the oils never leave my side. Petra explains that the oils have specific properties to improve many different health conditions and also have electrical frequencies to enhance our own body's frequency.
Greg and Pam are very encouraging. They tell me about their experiences when Greg nearly died a few years ago with Guillain Barre Syndrome. He was critically ill in intensive care and at around 10.45am one Sunday morning he surprised doctors by making a quick and miraculous recovery. Greg and Pam later found out that members of their church group attended a combined gathering where everyone prayed for Greg between 10.30 and 10.45am. Although Greg's initial recovery was swift, he spent the next three years battling the after effects of his illness. As a last resort he turned to Petra who identified many imbalances in his blood results. A few months of Petra's treatment enabled a very strong recovery.
At the end of the two weeks it's time for me to leave Petra. I'm scared. For these past weeks the loving care she has given me is beyond words. Physically, emotionally and spiritually this beautiful woman has nursed me back on the road towards health. Tirelessly she has tested, re-tested and treated my physical body. Emotionally she supported me, guided me and encouraged me to be positive. Each day she prayed with me for healing.
"How can I ever thank you enough?' I tell her. 'You're amazing."
"You don't need to thank me. You just get well."
Looking back at this time I see the importance of never giving up and just how important it is to keep trying, to listen to and follow your instincts as much as possible. If I had not seen Petra I have no doubt I would have died. Many months later when I was out of the woods Petra told me she believed I was only days away from dying. I completely agreed with her. Some may feel this is a worrisome statement but I felt a sense of relief that someone understood the dire situation I was in, whilst most

dismissed my concerns and told me I had anxiety. In years to come I am to learn there are not only hundreds, but thousands of people in this exact same situation, desperately ill and told it's all in their head; hypochondriacs suffering from some sort of syndrome, or possibly anxiety, maybe depression. Anything but the illness which has become an epidemic all around the world, the disease which I learn too many health professionals deny because they are unable to detect the disease with outdated testing methods being used.

4 Floating on a Sea of Uncertainty

Over the next six weeks my girls and I stay with my birth mother and her husband. Taking me shopping and helping me look after my girls, during this difficult time, their help is greatly appreciated. During one of our outings at the shops I barely have the strength to walk. I look at my girls. I cling on to every small thing I can give them even if it is just a smile. I look at my mother, so seemingly composed and strong. The pain of what it must be like to lose your child tears through me. I understand now what happens to people when they just shut off. Shut off their feelings. Shut off their heart. I can understand how losing a child could leave you totally empty. Unable to give. Nothing to give. Just numb.

When I was eighteen I knew I could look for my birth mother, but I had no burning desire to do so. It was a few years later at twenty-two that something urged me to look for her. I thought it would be fun to see what she looked like and if I had any sisters or brothers. I wasn't sure where to start, but the phone book seemed like a good place. I found a listing for adoption services and to my surprise within a couple of weeks I received a letter with my mother's contact details. Excitedly I wrote her a letter.

Soon after I received a small parcel. Opening it quickly I read the enclosed letter. My mother briefly explained a few mistakes that she had made when she was seventeen years old, which led to my arrival. Closely I examined the photos of my mother, her husband and my two sisters. I found a little resemblance, mainly in our eyes, but they are all dark haired and average height. I am tall and blonde. It seems I take after my father whose name my mother said she cannot give me. I didn't know why, but I had a deep sinking feeling in my stomach. Something didn't feel right. I ignored those feelings and happily continued examining the photos.

My mother and I wrote to each other over the next few months and she invited me to come and stay. My partner Mike was very busy with work, and I was reluctant to go on my own. My mother encouraged me to come anyway and we made plans, setting a date for the trip. As the time to leave neared, I became very excited and quite nervous. Finally I was on the train heading north. With a long trip ahead I tried to relax and make myself comfortable. I was happy to be distracted, invited to join a group of people on their way to a function.

"So where are you off to?"

"I'm going to meet my birth mother for the first time," I tell.

"You must be excited?"

"Very. But the closer we get the more nervous I'm becoming," I admit.
In the train watching the countryside go by I'm starting to feel slightly ill. Maybe some food will make me feel a bit better. I take a bite of an apple but put it aside. I notice myself becoming very twitchy. I can't help wriggling and tapping my fingers. I look at the photos in my hand. The minutes seem to be taking so long, but finally we grow near. We pass houses dotted here and there along the countryside. Soon they are lined up nicely beside each other as we enter the township.
A booming voice over the loud speaker alerts passengers we will be arriving in five minutes. I keep looking ahead as best I can. I see the station. I'm so excited and nervous. The train slows and I scan the people on the platform. I see her as the train passes. Our eyes meet for a split second. By the time the train comes to a stop I'm at one end of the platform and she is at the other. Feeling as though I'm in a movie, we walk towards each other looking over and around other people's heads. Finally, in the middle of the platform we embrace. We are both overjoyed and tearful at the same time.
I soon meet my stepsisters and my mother's husband. I am welcomed openly into the family. We discover many similarities and amazing coincidences. It turns out that my sisters also grew up with horses and went to pony club. When my mother was pregnant with me in Brisbane she lived with her brother just a few kilometres from where I grew up. Later my mother tells me about the skating rink where she met her husband.
"You have to be kidding? I used to go there every weekend when I was young," I exclaim.
"Well guess what? We later moved to the Gold Coast near where you are living now," my mother says.
How very bizarre. Somehow, without knowing it I've been following in my mother's footsteps my whole life.
I spend a nice week with my new family. Meeting my mother seems like meeting a long-lost aunt. There doesn't seem to be a profound heart felt connection between us, but there is certainly a connection, a feeling of deep familiarity. We build a fairly strong relationship over the following years visiting each other once or twice a year. Enjoying holidays together. My adopted family accept her as one of their own, the same way the rest of her family did me. Once I had children though, everything changed. I changed. I felt a strong need to know more of the circumstances surrounding my birth, particularly my father. This did not go well. What my mother told me was very different to what my aunt told me. This led

to more confusion and despair. Despite my efforts the small amount of information I had about my father was not enough to find him. I was very frustrated and angry, but eventually I came to the conclusion that my father could find me if he wanted to. During this difficult time, though I hadn't seen my mother for a number of years, she said she was still there for me and loved me. I realised I needed to appreciate that. Even so, our relationship was never the same.

Now I have new hurdles to deal with. I still wonder if I will get through each day. Very slowly I continue improving. My reactions after eating continue to be severe, but gradually I'm able to do more. I force myself to eat higher carbohydrate foods which I react to badly, but my joy seeing the numbers on the scales slowly growing higher is worth it. My mother is happy with the results and encourages me to keep at it. My belly is so distended it almost looks like I'm six months pregnant. Still sickly thin I know I look a mess. I try to hide myself behind loose clothing, but in the unbearable summer heat I finally give in, no longer caring what I look like. We're living in a small seaside village. Apart from the busy noisy port nearby it's a very pretty area. I'm relieved when my girls make friends with some nice kids. To see them enjoying themselves and having fun again. We meet the neighbours. Richard next door works at the port and spends most of his time off working on his own boat, which he has just built. Katie and her daughter over the road welcome us over for a swim in her pool any time we like. For this I am deeply grateful. I don't think she or anyone will ever realise how much relief it is for me when I am in the water, the incredible ease in my body.

It's the start of the year and Jemma attends the local high school, while Lily begins at the primary school. Thankfully they settle in really well. I feel sad I'm no longer home-schooling my girls but at the same time it's a relief while I'm so unwell. I do what I can to fill in my days. I feel caught between two worlds. I can't bear sitting still, but I don't have the energy or strength to do much. My blood tests show high levels of the stress hormone cortisol. I can feel the adrenalin constantly pumping through my body making me feel extremely anxious. Thankfully it's less than 100 metres to the beach. A walk I can manage now. I often float about in the water, wearing a long-sleeved shirt and long pants to avoid the deadly jellyfish which inhabit these waters at this time of year. Walking slowly back along the pathway in between the houses, all wet and bedraggled, I can't help being conscious of what a sickly sorry sight I must be.

My mother gives me a beautiful blanket she has knitted. At times there are moments of connection. A deep connection. She talks about feeling in a way she hasn't done for years, implying a deep happiness. But those moments seem to disappear as quickly as they come. She usually has a lot of time to herself and finds it difficult having us stay for an extended period. She makes it clear that she just won't be able to cope if we stay for long so I try to give her plenty of space. This is difficult as I feel a strong desire for her company and support. Sitting outside on the patio I return a wave to Richard busy building his boat.

Staying in contact with Petra she provides invaluable support and advice over the phone. She encourages me to have regular blood tests, which she combs through checking to see how my treatment may need to change. Finally my results are showing there is something wrong. The doctor is very concerned about my liver and advises that I should have a scan and possibly a biopsy. I find this all quite strange. For months I've been running around to so many medical and natural health practitioners desperately trying to find out what is wrong and my blood tests seemed okay. Now I'm finally starting to feel better and my tests are saying otherwise. I presume the release of toxins from my liver are now showing up in my blood. Though I'm still scared I have complete faith in the treatment Petra is giving me and I know it's working well. There's no way in the world I'm going to change anything or have any other invasive tests. I just know my body wouldn't handle it. Diligently I follow Petra's instructions. Bit by bit, I continue to improve.

I'm also receiving homeopathic treatment from a lovely man named Tim. At times, well most of the time I'm in despair especially not knowing what is wrong. Spending hours supporting me and discussing my symptoms, Tim works hard to find a remedy to match my mental, emotional and physical symptoms. Giving the body a dose of something similar to the condition it is experiencing, homeopathics work to activate your body's own self-healing mechanisms. I value practitioners like Tim, especially in this difficult time.

Caught in the same situation as so many people, I've been on a rollercoaster ride of ill-health for so many years, but now there seems to be no up-side of this ride and no stop button. I know many people experience similar things, with no answers and no relief. I'm just so thankful I've been able to find these practitioners who go way above and beyond their duty of care, their treatment and support helping me to get through each day.

Evenings are still a nightmare. The time I hate the most. Tossing and turning, unable to sleep. Going for a walk to the beach in the morning helps to lift my spirit but I find it very difficult to enjoy anything while feeling so awful all the time. Sitting on the patio, Richard and I say hello. He moves between the shed and his boat, sawing, hammering, varnishing and gluing. I make light conversation so I'm not just sitting awkwardly watching. With an offer to come and look at his work Richard opens the gate and guides me up the short ladder onto the boat. I compliment him on his beautiful work and admire the vibrant rich blue carpet, highlighting the varnished timber trim.

Over the weeks Richard and I talk a lot and I'm very grateful for his company.

"Every time you feel bad, you've just got to say to yourself, 'I'm strong and there's nothing wrong with me.' You can't let it beat you," he encourages.

Whether I believe it or not just his support makes me feel stronger and helps me to trust that I will get through this. I can't help but notice what a strong well-built man Richard is. I almost feel stronger just being around him. I spend a couple of hours enjoying his company while doing my little bit to help, then escape the heat in my neighbour Katie's pool. I relish every moment as the water soothes and nurtures my body. I find myself most days either in the pool, having a short walk to the beach, or at Richard's place watching him work on his boat, grateful for the company and temporary moments of relief. While I have been happy in my own company and quite a loner for many years, in this delicate state I notice a desperation for the company of others, easing the constant deep sense of fear within.

5 The Eye of the Storm

We've been here for six weeks now. My mother helps me look for an apartment or house nearby. I'm relieved to find a duplex a few blocks away. Still very unwell I'm worried about how I will cope. I find myself struggling to look after myself and my girls on my own. My mother wants to do all she can to support me but she also needs her free time and independence. Other than a trip to the shops once a week and church on Sunday I don't see her much. I'm needing more from her than she is able to give me. There is a deep part of me that yearns for a warm connection with my mother but a lifetime has separated us. She is no longer the person she was. Nor am I.

One afternoon I call my mother and ask her to take me to the doctor for a check-up as the pains I often get in my chest and left arm are very strong. Unfortunately she is unable to take me. I feel very disappointed, but I have just begun driving again so I take myself to the nearest hospital. I'm reassured when the ECG results come back fine, but the doctors are very worried about my overall state of health and wary of letting me leave. I still have a flicker of hope they will give me some answers but my condition baffles them. I tell them I've had all the tests under the sun and reassure them I've been having a lot of treatment so as long as my heart is okay I will manage.

Being in this new house is not going well. Jemma is not coping. Suddenly she has found herself to be the strongest and most capable person in the house. As a young teenager this is all too overwhelming. Lily a couple of years younger has a sense of security knowing that even though Jemma is unhappy she will always look out for her. Jemma is incredibly unhappy and agitated. I feel like I'm losing her and I'm very worried. I'm only just struggling to get through and don't feel I can give my girls anything more. I prevent them from going outside to see the boys who have begun to hang around. I hold them as much as possible tightly under my broken wings.

Before I became unwell our lives weren't perfect. We certainly had our share of problems, but they were vibrant and full of joy and happiness. Despite making some nice friends we are miserable. I don't remember a time in my life when I've ever felt so bleak. We miss our home, our community, our dear friends and the people and places we were so accustomed to. The little day-to-day routines and ways that made up our lives, giving wonderful feelings of familiarity are gone.

Quantum Health

Uncertain of how much health I will regain I wonder if we will ever be able to make a return home. When I receive calls from friends back home I'm inconsolable. I never realised just how deeply the people and places around us make up such a large part of who we are. I do not want to lose that part of myself. Though I have many people who I hold dear, I'm aware now of a small part of me has been fearful of allowing myself to be too close to people, for fear of losing them. I realise how limiting that fear has been for me and how much I need and want to be close to my loved ones.

An unexpected yet pleasant surprise is our neighbour Peter over the road. He introduces himself, his wife and their young daughter. Somehow he seems familiar. It turns out he is the brother of one of our home-schooling friends from back home. Not only have we met before, but we have spent a Christmas together. He insists we must come over and assures us he is always there if we need anything. This is a lovely blessing and gives me an incredible sense of comfort. I also see how much the girls appreciate being so openly welcomed and what a positive effect a connection with their friends back home has on them.

I join a Tai Chi class where I'm welcomed with open arms. I've never done this form of exercise before but anything to get out of the house and connect with people. I try to ignore the agonising discomfort in my body as I focus on the exercises. While the slow gentle and tranquil movements of Tai Chi are used to enable harmony in mind and body, I don't feel at all harmonious or tranquil. I do love though being with such a wonderful group of supportive women. They remind me that it's normal to need and want support and company. Their relaxed fun nature reminds me so much of my friends back home. One of the women gives me her number and says to call her if I need anything. I don't think I will need to, but the offer is worth more than I can tell her. Despite my constant struggle for health my sense of self is beginning to return.

Richard lends me his bike so I can ride down and visit. I take it easy, but after being so unwell even just gliding along slowly with the wind in my hair is wonderful. He is a continual source of strength and support. Every time he goes shopping or into town to pick up any bits or pieces for his boat I join him. As a single man who usually keeps to himself he seems to enjoy my company as much as I enjoy his. In a small village rumours are created and spread very quickly. Occasionally I hear whispers about Richard and I always being together. I guess that is understandable as we *are* together every day. When friends drop over to visit Richard I am there. Going to the shops I am there. In his boat I am there. Under different circumstances you never know what could develop but Richard is a gentleman and in my current state of health he asks for no more than friendship.

After helping on the boat for weeks I think I can almost class myself as first mate now. I climb the ladder with Richard following behind. "People must be thinking all sorts of things,' I laugh, 'with us spending hours here in your boat together."

"They can think what they like. Let's see if this is the right size. You can be extremely useful here. Just help me put this into place if you will."

Lying on a mattress in the berth we reach upwards pressing some carpet into place and rubbing out any bumps. After lying in silence for quite some time we look at each other and laugh. Once a few measurements are taken we go down to the shed. I help while he saws a piece of wood to the correct shape. Back to the boat again we confirm it fits well and then it's back to the shed for varnishing. I find this all very tiring but rewarding. I feel continuously exhausted, but I feel that way even if I do nothing. Worse though is the heat. Sitting in a chair I spray myself with water. I pick a grassy spot to lie down as awful sensations sweep over my body. I go over to Katie's pool for some relief. Having something to take interest in and these connections with people, no matter how brief, are so important providing something to look forward to in the day.

It's so frustrating and terrifying still not knowing what's wrong with me but each day I find myself able to do a little more and walk a little further. I'm glad I'm feeling a bit stronger, for I now have another challenge to face. Watching the television I see the eye of a cyclone building and heading straight towards us. Each day is difficult enough without having to deal with this!

It's the day before the cyclone. I find myself alone with my girls preparing to fend for ourselves. My mother has gone to stay with my sister. I'm terrified. Images of our roof being ripped off race through my mind. Being so unwell I've already been in a constant state of fear each day and night. Now I'm terrified. Not just for myself but for my girls.

"I don't know what to do in a cyclone," I think to myself. "Maybe we are supposed to get in the bath under a mattress. Maybe under the bed?" I look upwards raising my arms to the sky, "How much more am I supposed to take?" My anxiety levels are huge and my condition worsens. "I'm sure animals just drop dead," I tell myself, "under this much stress."

It's comforting when neighbours come to check up on us. Peter over the road is happy to help in any way. A lady a few doors down, who works with the weather bureau comes to update me, and I'm grateful for an offer to stay with them if need be. Richard isn't too fussed. He won't mind if his little old shack blows away. He wants to build a new house anyway. Later that day I receive a message from my sister asking if we are coming over. Joining my mother, sisters and the rest of the family, I'm relieved to take shelter there.

The cyclone passes during the night. Thankfully most areas don't have too much damage. A lot of debris and fallen trees but nothing too bad. The girls and I return to our house. With no power there is no refrigeration, or fans to escape the sweltering heat which seems to pierce every cell in my body aggravating my condition. I'm worried about our food supply. To regain my health and minimise my severe reactions the only foods I've been eating over the past few months are fresh fruit, vegetables and protein. I have tinned food, but to my relief Peter brings over a large esky and informs me that the shop nearby has ice. I cannot thank him enough. The power shortage lasts for three days. Each day is extremely difficult but somehow we manage to get through.

I've not heard from my mother during this time. While I'm disappointed I no longer try to make our relationship anything more than it is, and accept things as they are. A while after the power comes back on I receive a message. It's my mother. I find it hard to understand what she's saying. I think she's apologising for not seeing me or checking on how we're going with no power. I don't want to feel needy anymore and I don't want to cause any conflict. "It's fine," I reply. As it turns out I have misread the message. Later in the day my mother is here. Holding a piece of paper in front of me in anger, she has typed and printed out all of our text messages word for word.

"Here you said 'that's fine' and down here you said 'that's fine'. What did you mean by that?"

I am bewildered! With exasperation I try to explain, "What I meant is, it doesn't matter what happens, I am fine with it." I realise that none of my words are being heard or understood. My mother becomes even more upset and tries to explain why she is angry.

"Are you fine with that?" she asks me.

I am really bewildered. Her angry voice becomes like a distant humming and I can barely hear what she is saying. I feel my whole nervous system, my whole body, shaking, jittery and fragile. I am unwell. I am weak. I am broken. "No, I mean, whether you come and see me or if you don't, that is fine."

She leaves abruptly. All I can think is that I have to get out of here. I have always been very proud to be strong and able to handle anything that comes my way, but for the first time I know what people mean when they say their nerves are shot.

As the cyclone moves away the weather clears but some waves remain. A rare thing with islands and reef preventing most swell from hitting the coastline.

"Look mum, we've got surf!!' my girls exclaim. 'Come on, let's go! Come for a surf with us mum."

I really don't see how I could possibly survive it. I know I shouldn't go and try to put up all sorts of reasons why not, but eventually I give in with a touch of rebellious excitement. What on earth am I doing? I barely have the strength to carry the board down to the beach, let alone go out in the water. Oh well, even if I die now at least I'm doing something enjoyable and I can't resist having a little fun with my girls. We need some sort of joy in our lives. I ignore the distress in my body. Just watching the girls laughing and enjoying themselves pushes me on, helping me find strength while the water cools and eases my body.

I try to keep the girls close to me as the water surges around us. The sea is very messy and choppy. "Paddle over here. Stay close to me," I insist. These waters are new to me. I can't tell if there are any rips or undertows. We are all happy to catch a couple of waves. I struggle to my feet and ride one wave a short distance. The wind and water is washing us all over the place. I suddenly become aware of what a mistake this may be. If something happens I won't have the strength to deal with it as I normally could. The current sweeps us closer to the rocks. "Come on, we'd better go in now," I call out.

I'm relieved when we make it to shore safely. The surfing wasn't a huge success but just being out there in a cyclone swell, even if it wasn't really all that big gives us all a sense of accomplishment. Most of all we had fun. And even more importantly I am there for them. I suffer the consequences after surfing and for the next few days my muscles are tingling, burning and cramping even more than usual. It's very difficult to sleep at all but it was worth it.

6 Born to Be

When you are extremely unwell you do not have the strength to hold on to anything that is no longer good for you. You find that you *have* to hold on with all your might to the things that are. For the first time in my life I am clearly able to distinguish between the two. I begin to find a strength within that I never imagined I had. I find myself enduring things I never imagined possible. I think about my close family and friends. Now more than ever I need their love and support. I need their nurturing. I realise deep within myself how to fully open my heart and let people close to me. I begin to see clearly where people fit into my life.
I have never felt so alone. I know my birth mother has given me as much as she can. Most importantly she introduced me to Petra, who saved my life. My birth family have been good to my girls and I, having us stay with them, but despite some strong similarities our ways and expectations are extremely different. I realise how strongly the environment in which you live influences your life and beliefs, your way of thinking and living.
It's time to go home. I need to go home. My girls need to go home. Dad was almost fifty when he adopted me. He and my step mother, now in their eighties, recently moved into an aged home. Dad calls regularly and I try not to cry when I hear his voice. I don't want him to worry about me more than he already does. "I'm slowly getting better, Dad," tears stream down my face as I try so hard to have a normal voice.
"Is there anything I can do for you?"
Despite his intentions there's nothing he can do.
"Just hearing your voice is enough," I cannot control my sobs.
"Come on now, you're alright."
"Yes, I'm alright Dad," I say trying to hide my despair. "I'm just so happy to talk to you. You have always been so good to me. I love you so much."
"I love you too Di," he reassures me in his familiar deep, warm voice.
"I'm so glad you are my Dad. I'm so glad you adopted me."
"I'm glad too, but I didn't like it when you always ran off down the horse paddock though."
I giggle in between tears. Dad always reminds me about that. If I was angry or upset I would take off down to my horse paddock and sit with Cobba. Sometimes I would lie across his back laying my head on his soft rump as he walked around in the moonlight. If Dad came looking for me I would often hide up a tree. "We're coming home Dad! Probably next week"

I muster up my strength and start making arrangements. I say my goodbyes and thankyous to all who have helped me and nursed me through this time. I feel sad to say goodbye to Richard. While he plays it cool I can see his disappointment. All the same the quicker I can get out of here the better. I talk to my mother and her husband, and tell them how grateful I am for the help they have given me. I'm quite surprised by the response. My mother is very upset we're going, to the point she seems quite irrational. I'm confused. In the past six weeks we've had such little connection. One minute she is angry, the next she is upset, saying she doesn't know what else she could have done for me. I'm really confused, but I know that all I can do is look after myself and my girls. I do not have anything to give her. I cannot support her. I need to go.

I worry a little about the drive ahead but the cool air conditioning and the vibration of the car soothe my body. My concentration on the road takes my attention away from how I'm feeling. In fact I find driving more relaxing than lying down. I joke with myself that maybe I should be a truck driver. I could just drive and drive all day. I call Dad on one of our stops to let him know that we are about half way.

"You be careful driving, won't you?"

Dad has always been a worrier. I guess that has been since his first wife, my adopted mother, died when I was three and a half years old. Dad's second wife, who he married when I was five had also lost her husband when her children were young. During my childhood she was hospitalised a number of times receiving shock treatment in an attempt to improve her mental health. For as long as I can remember she was on such medication as Valium. I never really noticed that she had much of a problem apart from the times she was hospitalised. I just didn't like it when she was always 'vagued out' and not really there. We had never been especially close but she was a very good, caring and devoted mother and wife. Apart from when she was hospitalised she was always there for me if I needed her and she looked after my sister and I well. As an adult I was quite surprised and happy to learn that before she even met my father she had wanted to adopt more children. Somehow there was an awakening within me when I learned this.

Arriving in Brisbane we head straight to visit Mum and Dad. My appreciation for them has never been so deep. Sitting outside in the garden Dad snuggles me under his shoulder filling me with love and warmth. I rest my head on his chest. Despite his aging body becoming more frail, he still feels strong. His large hand holding mine reminds me of our evening walks when I was a child, strolling hand in hand. Mum and I embrace deeply. She tells me what a good girl I have always been. That is very nice of her considering all my mischievous behaviour and adventures as a child providing endless loads of muddy washing. Or maybe it's the dementia setting in. Either way we share a deep heartfelt love and respect. It's very special.

I'm beginning to see that despite the trauma I've experienced, I have been given more love, caring and understanding than some people receive in a lifetime, even from their biological family. As I grew up things were certainly not perfect, in fact there were plenty of problems but my parents were there for me, always doing the best they could, and their love for me was unconditional.

We head to Lennie and Barb's house to stay for a few days. The girls and I are relieved to feel so at home and welcomed. Lennie and I have been good mates since I was sixteen, close to thirty years now. He is like a brother. He is a brother. Our next stop on the way home is to my beautiful homebirth midwife Claire.

"Hello darling. You haven't been well. This is not good," she says in her French/Canadian accent as we all embrace. "And look at your two beautiful young women now."

Claire supported me during my first pregnancy and homebirth, guiding me and helping me to empower myself as a woman and mother. She explained that it is the mother who births the baby. The role of the midwife is to create a safe and protected space for the mother to do so. I love this wonderful woman, filled with wisdom and knowledge, sharing her natural and home remedies.

Before I fell pregnant I was seeing a German doctor, who used many natural therapies. His treatments and suggested dietary changes greatly improved my health in my early twenties. Using a Vega machine which monitors the electrical frequencies in the body he detected a number of allergies which he treated with the machine. When I became pregnant, I don't know where I got the idea, but I asked the doctor if he knew anything about homebirths. He gave me the number of a midwife from the Gold Coast Hospital who highly recommended it. I was impressed. If she recommended homebirth I decided it must be worthwhile. She gave me the contact details of the local homebirth group. Made up of numerous mothers and midwives they shared a wealth of information and their experiences discussing different options, techniques and

treatments. I did a lot of research which showed the rate of complications and caesareans is quite low in women who choose

homebirths. A number of reports found the drugs used to induce labour and for pain relief can cause complications. Looking at national statistics it seemed that homebirths are a very safe option, and considering I was only five minutes from the hospital I felt confident to plan a homebirth.
Early on in my pregnancy I pushed myself to go to work despite feeling terrible. That afternoon I had a threatened miscarriage. I never realised before how devastating this might be. I was terrified I would lose the baby. I went to bed and figured if I didn't move all would repair itself and the baby would be fine. I thank God all was fine and the rest of my pregnancy went smoothly. Claire lovingly supported me through the whole process with a long first stage in a birthing pool relaxing to my favourite meditative music. With the water a little cool Claire instructed me to hop out of the pool when second stage began.
"It's hurting," I complained.
"Yes, you're having baby," she replied in her nonchalant manner, to which I could not help but laugh.
With only a few pushes my precious Jemma arrived two and a half weeks early. I was thrilled and in awe of this beautiful birth. I feel a huge sense of accomplishment.
Over the next week Claire would come to check on Jemma and me each day. During the following months I'd ring her if I was worried about anything. Often she'd suggest a simple home remedy or a natural treatment which usually resolved the problem quickly. Occasionally she'd just say, "You know what to do darling."
Her confidence in me was so reassuring. But I certainly don't know what I need for myself now. Claire supports me with a craniosacral treatment. Gently holding the back of my head she uses barely noticeable movements to restore the natural position of the cranium, the bones of my head, and balance the rhythmic wave-like pulses that go through the cranium, spinal column, sacrum and the entire body. After a check-up she agrees my liver has been having a difficult time and is quite swollen. She gives me grape seed extract in case of parasites. It is also antibacterial, antiviral and anti-inflammatory and useful to cleanse the digestive system. I'm also given bentonite clay, which draws toxins from the body while the clay itself has a range of nutrients and an abundance of minerals, including calcium, magnesium, silica, sodium, copper, iron and potassium. Claire confirms the other herbs I am taking are good for my condition. "Maybe you should try the breathwork again," she suggests as we leave.

Quantum Health

My first experience with breathwork was a year after the birth of Jemma. Described as a powerful form of self-exploration and healing, there are many forms of breathwork which use one or a combination of breathing exercises, including gentle or forced breath, bodywork, shamanism, transpersonal psychology, talk, art, or music therapy and rebirthing techniques. Becoming a mother opened me up to a whole new world of experience. A side of myself I had shut down years before. Unlocking my heart to the deep love that I felt for my child, allowing myself to feel, meant also unlocking the grief and turmoil hidden within. I could have been diagnosed with post-natal depression, yet I knew I held unresolved grief which I needed to address. Counselling was helpful but I needed something more, something deeper. My counsellor referred me to a practitioner called Anne who uses very gently methods. During a session, Anne would simply lie me down on a mattress on the floor encouraging me to focus on my breath and the feelings in my body. At first it felt a little strange, but soon emotions would spontaneously come to the surface to be expressed and released providing a huge sense of relief, often followed by deep feelings of love.

For the first time in my life I learned how to listen to my body. To care for myself and respect my own feelings. It was wonderful. I learnt to allow my emotions, be they good or bad. I released a lot of anger, grief, turmoil and tears. It was very difficult at times but more than anything it was such a relief. The love and peace I felt was heavenly, even euphoric. Seeing Anne monthly or fortnightly during the next three years was a deeply healing time in my life.

After moving north I continued using the breath and meditation techniques. My passion for breathwork grew strong. I found myself wanting to do little else. I began to realise I was using breathwork and meditation as an escape from the 'real world' and even more feelings of grief held within. Doing so was having a detrimental effect. I became quite 'vagued out' which reminded me of my step mother when she was on Valium when I was a child, but I had learnt how to avoid pain without the drugs. My thoughts and awareness were so often drifting away to the feelings of love I had discovered within myself and in the past, but this state of vague, out-of-body blissfulness was keeping me out of touch with love and life in this physical world.

Now my passion for breathwork diminished. I focused more on day to day activities and being a mum and didn't do any breathwork for a few years. I realise now that learning a way to balance and integrate these learnings and practices into our daily life is the key.

7 The Breath of Life

Driving back to our home town is like being able to breathe again. The relief is enormous. Just sitting by the ocean watching the waves is deeply relaxing. A trip to the shops and I can't count the number of friends and familiar faces who stop to chat or say hello. It's heart-warming. I'm blessed to be part of this wonderful supportive community. Since having to sell our home to pay for medical bills, we are staying with our good friend Jim. He's a wonderful support and very understanding when it comes to health issues, one of the few who really gets it. Jim had a number of health problems many years ago and made a lot of changes to his diet to improve his health. He has read many books and is a wealth of information when it comes to living and eating naturally. Jim's diet consists mostly of fruit and vegetables. Working in the building industry he rides his bike to work each day, sometimes over twenty kilometres, and then labours all day. After the ride home he might go for a run along the beach on the soft sand or for a surf.

I see my dear friends Julie and Pete who are so incredibly caring and jovial, lifting my spirits higher than they've been in a very long time. I know I can talk to them about any and everything. They encourage me to come along to table tennis. Despite feeling jittery and weak I quietly push on, thriving on the jovial fun and rivalry. The agony and severe ill-health I still feel in my body daily is terrifying. To feel this way with no medical support or assistance, no one knowing what is wrong is horrendous.

Many people are simply unable to comprehend what I'm going through, just as I wouldn't have been able to understand it in the past. Well I still don't understand it but having just a few people who are able to sit beside me in the depths of this darkness is a precious gift. When you are in such a deep state of fear and agony you feel very alone, to the depths of your soul. To have someone meet you at that place, hold your hand with no judgement, no expectation, to simply be there, provides a deep sense of security for the soul, which in turn is very healing. In front of everyone I put on a smile and don't tell of the agony inside, day in day out. I know most people don't understand, nor can they do anything. Most of all if I can't feel 'normal' I want to be treated as though I am, not the sickly walking death that I've been.

My recovery over the following months is very slow. It's frustrating and unnerving not knowing what is wrong with me. I'm still having severe reactions after eating with agonising pain throughout my whole body, burning in my chest, and cramping and tingling in my muscles. I manage to function with little sleep. I have to just keep on pushing myself to get through each day. With determination I continue to put on weight and build my strength. Eating a large variety of food I discover that since my kidney and liver cleanses I no longer have any of my usual food allergies causing digestive problems, bloating, diarrhoea or asthma. I would prefer to have those reactions to food rather than the reactions I'm having now but still it's good to have another improvement in my health. My latest blood tests are showing my liver results have returned to normal which is certainly another good sign.

With my body in a continual state of stress I can easily notice the effect on my body when I'm upset. Just thinking about something that slightly upsets me, I feel a wave of adrenalin pump through my body increasing my already rapid heartbeat. It's awful. I begin to train my thoughts and focus my attention. I watch and observe what's happening in my body and mind. I'm able to distinguish clearly between feeling anxious because of the physical symptoms in my body, and feeling anxious because of my thoughts and emotions. If a thought upsets me I refuse it. I change that thought and focus on something positive, anything to ease my body. I'm always looking within myself to see if there's something I need to learn, or patterns that need changing. While this doesn't seem to ease my reactions after eating or my physical symptoms a great deal, I am regaining my emotional strength. I realise that despite the intense pain, anger or fear we may feel at times, it is vitally important for our physical, mental and emotional wellbeing to gain control over our thoughts and the way we respond and react to them.

I begin seeing another naturopath who uses a Vega testing machine as part of her treatment, which detects the frequencies of parasites, viruses, bacteria, held in the body. Amongst other things she treats me for parasites and warns that I may have a 'die off' and feel a little worse at first. Sure enough for the next day or two I feel terrible, but soon I begin to have slight improvement.

In this bizarre world of synchronicity two different people in one week tell me some amazing stories of healing by a man named Geoff. I wonder why I haven't heard of him before. Feeling hopeful and curious I make an appointment. He sits me down on a chair. Somehow, even with all my clothes on he can see everything that is happening in my body. The stress in my muscles and tendons. Ribs out of place. Old injuries. I'm dumbfounded. To my surprise he tells me some of this could have happened in the womb. He picks up a pen and directs it a couple of inches away from my body. He seems to be going from one point to another as though he's doing a dot to dot above my body. He works his way around my jaw, neck and down my arms, occasionally stopping to rub certain areas.

"That's sore isn't it? Yep," he says before I have a chance to reply, while I nod in agreement. He points the pen at me a few times then presses with his fingers on the same sore points. Moving his way up my body, he criss-crosses from my chest to my neck. I feel as though something is moving up my throat. I don't know what to do as this bizarre sensation almost overwhelms me. What's happening? I think. As Geoff points the pen at me, raising it higher it feels like I'm about to regurgitate something. As the sensation moves to the top of my throat it disappears. My eyes are full of tears. I don't know what has just happened. I feel like I've had some sort of huge emotional and physical release.

"All down your right-hand side here isn't good, is it?"

"I've had trouble down my right side for a long time,' I tell.

"I can see that. That's not the main cause though. Down here, that's pulling across here and affecting your stomach. That's sore there isn't it," he says pressing a point on the lower part of my ribs.

"Yes, very. I have all these really bad reactions after eating. I've been really sick."

"Mmm, I can see all the nerves there are inflamed."

Geoff has a good 'look' all around my lower chest and abdomen, feeling and pressing different points. I don't know what he is looking at or how he is seeing anything through my shirt. I am burning with curiosity.

"How can he see all this?"

"I just see it," he says, "I think you've got a stomach ulcer. I can help to relax things, but you will have to go to the doctor and get some medication. Geoff goes over my whole body pointing the pen at me, pressing different spots and moving my limbs around then asks me to stand up and have a walk around.

"Oh, I can hardly stand up," I say. "This is amazing. It feels so weird. I feel so relaxed."

As I move and stretch I feel like I could just slump down onto the ground. Like a switch of tension has been flicked off. Over the next day or two though I'm still having severe reactions after eating, I notice my sleep is less broken and I'm relieved to feel a little more relaxed. Another step forward.

The girls and I spend a fun weekend up the coast with Deb, Travis and their kids and I thank them so dearly for all the help and support they have given us while I've been unwell. While these horrid sensations are still in my body screaming at me trying to take my attention, I refuse to let it ruin my weekend. I'm doing everything I can to improve my health so for now I ignore them the best I can and clutch onto these joyful times. The next day we make our way home and I receive a call from my brother. Dad is in hospital. They are worried he won't make it through the night. Even if I did find the strength to make the drive back up the coast I don't have the strength to cope with losing Dad. Not yet. In the morning to my relief I find out he has made it through the night and all his vital signs have improved. Over the following weeks he makes a fairly strong recovery and returns to the aged hostel where the girls and I visit Mum and him regularly.

Still weary and struggling with my health I keep myself as busy as I can so I don't have to think too much about how I feel. Study and volunteer work fill in many hours but sitting in an office is something I've never wanted to do. Despite feeling horribly caged in it's one of the few things I can do while my health is not good. My thoughts keep wandering to breathwork. I completed the first unit of a Certificate IV a few years ago. Becoming a practitioner still crosses my mind but I wonder how on earth I can help other people if I can't even help myself. Regardless of my concerns breathwork seems to be my calling and I can't ignore it so I decide to throw myself in head first and commit to completing the course in the hope it will also help me.

With the girls cared for, I stay with my stepbrother Christian, and his wife Rose. The first training intensive is underway. At the beginning of each session we write down our intentions, set in a positive frame and in the present tense. Lying down we are guided into deep relaxation with beautiful calm music in the background. We are encouraged to allow any sensations, thoughts and feelings in our body, noticing them, but always bringing our awareness back to our body and our breath.

With breath sessions every day I set my intentions about what I would like to improve in my own life. Needless to say my intention is to heal.

"Well you have your intention, you *are* healing. And you might be healing for the next twenty years," my trainer says. "How do you want to be once you *have* healed?"

"I want to be strong and healthy." I reply.

The trainer explains how important it is to always look for the positive outcome.

Over and over every day I repeat to myself, "I intend to be really strong and healthy, I intend to be strong and healthy." I am wary of repeating my habit of using breathwork as an escape from what is actually going on in my life so I remind myself to focus on what I'm feeling, here and now. Acknowledging my feelings I bring my awareness back to my body and remember to breathe nice full relaxed breaths.

I go and see the doctor who treated Christian when he had a stomach ulcer a few years earlier. I'm hopeful I'll be able to take some medication and all will be better. Unfortunately testing for the bacteria that cause stomach ulcers proves negative. The doctor says my symptoms are pointing so strongly towards an ulcer that he's happy to prescribe the medication anyway. It does provide some relief with slight improvement of some of my digestive problems but not the outcome I'm hoping for. Disappointed, I wonder what I'm doing here. What on earth am I thinking this breathwork is going to do to help? What will ever help me?

With no answers and no other medical support when you're chronically unwell it is so easy to fall into despair and lose all hope of regaining health. This is a time when you need to dig deep and find somewhere within, the strength to hold on to your belief that you will get well.

Every day again and again I set my intentions during the breath sessions, "I intend to be really healthy, I intend to be strong and healthy." During the training I become good friends with the other trainee Miriam. While I experienced conflict with my older sister, she had a younger adopted brother, who she experienced conflict with. Despite our initial apprehension we form a strong sisterly bond laughing and giggling throughout our training. This turns out to be a healing gift for both of us and a great support during some unexpected difficulties during the training.

After each session we have paper and coloured pencils to draw any visions and thoughts we may have had. One day I draw an image of my body. Afterwards I realise I have drawn a black curving line of energy representing my spine. I wonder why I have drawn it black? Feeling this is not a good thing I try to rub it out, but I can't so I convince myself there's nothing wrong and it's a good thing. I have some interesting experiences and different sensations in my body during the sessions. No thunderbolts from the sky or miraculous instant healing but as can often happen after a breathwork session, over the next couple of weeks one of the major causes of my ill-health finally surfaces; an abscess develops on the gum above one of my teeth.

Eight years earlier after a filling I experienced extreme pain in that tooth. Ever since, I have known something wasn't right. I had it checked a couple of times over the years but I was told it was fine. I'd heard your teeth can have a big effect on your health and it did cross my mind to have the tooth taken out. But I decided it was nothing and my tooth was far too important to just go and get rid of it. Now though, I go straight to see my dentist with the intention of having it removed immediately if necessary. Luckily I met this dentist at a holistic dental conference twenty years ago and he recently began a practice close by. Up-to date with the latest research and practises in healthy dentistry, he is now confirming what my intuition told me. With removal of the tooth he informs me there was a very big abscess going right up into my sinus, it would have taken years to get this big, and it would have been poisoning me!

Each month I attend breathwork training intensives, sometimes taking the girls with me. I'm enjoying the opportunity to spend time with Christian and Rose. For over twenty years they've been practising Kirtan chanting and sacred ceremonies. Now each morning we collect flowers and carry out a ritual of devotion, chanting, playing guitar and harmonium, and as an offering provide a small meal, burning of incense, water and blowing of a conch shell. Chanting the mantras is mesmerising. Described as transcendental sound vibrations, they deliver the mind from material anxieties. I never knew I could sing before. I *couldn't* sing before, but somehow I have found my voice and I love it. To connect with spirit and sacred universal energy is very nourishing to the soul. I listen to Christian's voice reading the ancient sandskrit scriptures called the Upanisad, which speak of our difficulties in life only occurring because we have lost touch with our original pure consciousness. In that state we do not suffer birth, death, disease or old age.

Christian and Rose often take us to large gatherings and I'm mesmerised by the beautiful soft chanting. We all receive a delicious vegetarian meal and luscious dessert. The last half of the night is upbeat, the singing and dancing loud and joyful, the atmosphere now electric and entrancing. The connection I feel with these people despite many of them being strangers, is a connection of the soul. It doesn't matter your personality, what you like or don't like, everyone here has the intention to find fulfilment and oneness at a deep level. A connection with the divine, which is incredibly healing for mind, body and soul.

The next day Christian tells me they are going to see a Chinese doctor who has been highly recommended and asks if we would like to come along. Still desperate to get well I'll try anything. We arrive at a small house filled with Chinese people. The lounge room is a combined waiting and treatment room. In one corner herbs are in boxes, on shelves and hanging from the ceiling. Two ladies stand at a bench sorting herbs which have been prescribed by the doctor into portions then into bags. Many people are waiting while the doctor treats each patient at a desk at the side of the room. As my turn arrives he asks me to sit down. Taking my hand he gently feels my pulse. After only one or two minutes he says something I presume in mandarin to his daughter who tells me that my stomach is fine and I can eat anything. I nod in sheer amazement. I can't help laughing. Over the past year or two the reactions I've had after eating have been a nightmare. How on earth did he know? I can't believe how incredibly accurate he is. With each one of us he detects our physical problems and also describes in detail our personality traits despite the fact that we have not said a word to him other than hello. I am in awe of this amazing medicine man. The ladies at the counter weigh the correct amount of each herb and invite Lily and Jemma to help mix and separate them into portions before scooping into paper bags.

At home we boil up our teas. I find them very strong, but with a lot of honey they are bearable. Poor Rose is nauseous each time she drinks her potion.

"Oh, that looks like a beetle," I say looking at my tea.

"It *is* a beetle," laughs Jemma in horror.

Oh well, I will do whatever I can to regain my health. Over the following weeks I notice more improvements but once again it's not the answer of all answers I was hoping for. Jemma on the other hand, though she didn't really have any noticeable problems, rather than sleeping in and waking tired, she now wakes up quite early full of energy.

During the breath sessions I continue focusing on my intentions to be really healthy. This time I decide to up the ante. "I intend to be and feel really healthy, surfing, running and swimming again." This is a big call for I'm unsure if I will ever be able to do much activity again. I have no immediate or dramatic improvements, but as time goes on my body continues to grow stronger and I notice how much more energy I have. Little by little I begin paddling out on my board. It's blissful to be out in the water again, even just sitting there as the swells pass under me. The constant movement and coolness of the water eases my body. It feels like I'm living again. I find I need to take it easy though, because I'm a wreck for a couple of days after surfing and the increased buzzing and tension in my muscles makes it even harder for me to sleep.

It's now almost a year since my treatment with Petra. Jemma's surfing is improving and she's very keen to be in the water. Though she's becoming more confident out the back in the bigger waves she still likes to have me there by her side. I've missed so much of my girls' lives over the past year or so, caught up in my own struggles that I want to do as much as I can with them.

"Are you coming surfing with me again Mum?" pleads Jemma.

Not wanting to overdo things I say no, but soon cave in. I encourage and support the girls and attempt catching a few waves myself.

"Look, dolphins," calls Jemma.

Joyfully we watch as the dolphins swim and jump out of the waves towards us. Their silvery grey bodies glide through the water beneath pushed along by the surge of the wave, rising here and there around us, the sound of air gushing through their blowholes as they take a breath. I'm so filled with joy to be in the ocean with my girls again and so incredibly blessed to be having this amazing experience.

I spend many hours on my own, but as I'm learning during this process of healing, it's deeply important at times to feel a part of life and the world around. Even if only for just a short while, it takes you out of the inner world of suffering you may be experiencing, giving a feeling or glimmer of normality and hope. As I am soon to discover, not only is this helpful for our general state of mind, but it also triggers a very powerful process of healing on many deep levels.

8 The Breath of Heaven

Day by day Dad is becoming weaker, his life force disappearing. We visit him regularly. His large strong frame is now thin and fragile. But he's just as demanding as he has always been and stubbornly determined to hold on to as much independence as he can. As the nurse says it's probably an attribute that has helped him to live such a long generally healthy and independent life. Having been in a very powerful position for most of his working life Dad is accustomed to people following his orders. I'm sure the nurses and staff find him quite difficult at times but they are also softened by his warm caring, his dry and witty sense of humour, and the many compliments he gives them.

The family have known for a couple of weeks that Dad does not have long to live. Boxing Day afternoon I receive a call. There's no doubt he will pass away soon. This time I am ready. I feel strong enough now and don't want to see Dad struggle any more. I feel almost happy that he'll finally be able to move on. Along the highway driving down the range the dark and stormy clouds part just enough to let rays of sunlight illuminate the most magnificent rainbow. It stretches across an incredibly beautiful scene below with miles of rolling green fields beside the ocean. I'm surprised to find myself smiling and feeling happy.

On my arrival I brace myself. I take a deep breath and join my brother and sister by Dad's side. His face is drawn and barely recognisable. I'm informed he is dropping in and out of consciousness, partly due to the high doses of morphine, easing the pain of his broken rib after a fall last week. Errol, Dad's biological son, is more than twenty years older than me and a tower of strength taking charge of anything that needs to be done. We sit by Dad's side for hours taking turns to hold his hands and comfort him. He's unable to talk but it does seem at times he is aware of our presence. We bring Mum in to sit with him for a short time and then take her back to her room. Over the past six months or so her dementia has increased as quickly as Dad's health has decreased.

I notice Dad's breathing and what's happening in his body, the cycles of intensity and calmness. Every five or ten minutes a wave of tension comes over his body. His breathing becomes rapid and he is extremely anxious, seemingly in pain. After a few minutes his body eases, his breath relaxes and he becomes calm again. This continues all through the night. I cannot believe how similar his breathing patterns are to those of a woman in labour. Having completed most of my breathwork training I can't help being curious about what's happening in his body and his soul.

By 4 am I've had a few ten or fifteen minute naps with my head on Dad's bed. It feels like this might go on for days. I tell my brother I might just lie down for a short rest. He encourages me to have a drink and a little walk around. One of the nurses does her usual check on Dad. "You can go now Arthur," she says.

I guess that's something we've all been thinking but haven't said. My brother, sister and I talk to him and tell him he can go now. It doesn't feel quite right. I have a niggling feeling I shouldn't be telling Dad what to do! I can hear his voice in my mind, "I will go when I'm good and ready." Thinking about it for a minute I change what I'm saying. "It's okay if you go now Dad. We all know you have given us everything you can possibly give us. You have been such a fantastic Dad and we all love you so much. We're all fine."

To my surprise within minutes I notice Dad's breathing patterns change. He is no longer breathing into the lower parts of his chest. His breath is only going into his throat and the very top of his chest. His body cannot be getting enough oxygen now. I point this out to my brother and the nurse, who asks my sister to come in after a short walk. We call our other sister Judith in New Zealand. She tells him how much she loves him as Dad takes his last breath.

We comfort each other and a few tears come to my eyes. I wipe them away and swallow. I don't want to cry. I have done enough crying in recent times. I want to be strong. I need to be strong. I do not need to grieve for I know Dad is with me. In every cell of my body I will hold his love within me. Always. I make a strong conscious effort to transform any feelings of grief, into relief and happiness. I want to celebrate his life and his passing with joy. He would like that.

My sister and I bring Mum back in to sit with Dad. We tell her that he has passed away. She doesn't remember or understand much at all these days but Dad is the one thing she does know. It's very painful seeing her grief. We comfort her while she sits with him. When she begins to doze off we take her back to her room to lie down. An hour or two later on waking she's perfectly happy with no recollection of the evening before. The staff assist her with her daily routine and she carries on as if nothing has happened.

It's now daylight and I just want to go home and be with my girls. I promise Errol I will stop if I need to rest. I drive for over an hour before I realise I really do need to sleep so I stop for a rest. I know my body is going to be shattered for days after missing a night's sleep. It would be nice if life could just stop for us until we are in a place where we feel ready for everything, but it just doesn't. This is when life calls for complete surrender. Letting go of everything you thought was or should be. Finding the deepest trust in the universe or God. Finding, as hard as it may be, the trust that he/she has got this and everything is happening when and where it is meant to.

9 The Ride of My Life

Four weeks of holidays to go and the girls are keen to be at the beach nearly every day. Over the four months or so since having my bad tooth removed my energy levels have continued to rise. I'm surfing fairly regularly and find I'm not 'crashing' as much afterwards. Each day though is still a struggle. The burning sensations after eating, muscle cramps and twitches, aches, and heart palpitations. Night sweats. Jittery shakiness and my whole nervous system still shot. Brain fog and short-term memory loss. I continue to get by with little sleep. If I manage to get five or six hours a night I'm happy. I try to listen to my body regularly and pay attention to how I'm feeling as I would normally do in a breath session, but all the beautiful meditation, relaxation and breathing techniques I've used in the past give my physical body no relief.

I take the herbal teas for kidney and liver cleansing religiously each day and continue to keep busy which helps take my mind off how bad I feel all the time. It's exhausting and even when I do rest, I don't *feel* rested so I just keep on going. I have become fed up with worrying about the heart palpitations. Now out surfing when my heart is jumping, racing and skipping all over the place I can't be bothered with it. That happens a lot when I'm doing nothing anyway so I just keep on at a leisurely pace doing what I'm doing. I'm starting to feel a little invincible. If I was going to die I would have done it by now. And after all I've been through over the past year and a half my heart is still beating hard and strong.

So surf and surf we go. Being in the water soothes my body. It is heavenly. Every time I think I won't be able to do more I find that I can.

"Go Jem, paddle hard. Go," I encourage as I see a good wave coming.

Happily I watch her take off on the wave gliding along. "Did you see that one mum!" she yells as she paddles back out.

"Yeah, that was a beauty. That would have been one of your longest rides ever, wouldn't it?"

"Yeah, one of," she beams.

"Come on Lil, catch a greenie," I say.

In between wipe-outs Lily is having a great time too, occasionally catching waves all the way in to the beach.

Angourie Point is a world-famous surf break which runs along the northern side of the picturesque Angourie headland. On the southern side is Angourie Bay, or Back Beach as most surfers call it. I've never surfed the point. The first time I came here I saw someone caught at 'Life

and Death', a rock ledge at the end of the break. If you get caught there when the swell is big it really *is* a matter of life and death. Thankfully the guy survived his experience with no major injuries but that was enough to put me off. Now though, my confidence is growing. The surf is nice and small and I wonder if I should give it a go.
"Hey, are you coming out?" says Cathy, a long-time local.
"Mmm, I've been thinking about it, but I've never surfed here. I saw someone caught at life and death a few years ago."
"It's fine today. You won't have any problems at all. Come on."
Following Cath I paddle out warily.
"See, easy as that," she says as we get out there.
"That *was* easy. Thanks heaps."
There's a lot of competition at most good surf breaks and Angourie is no exception. I see a couple of faces I recognise. I'm happy to sit back patiently and see if a wave comes my way. I hope I can at least get one wave and assert my position out here. I paddle for a couple but they suck up very quickly so I pull back. Another wave comes in the right spot for me. I just have to go for it. I'm a bit slow getting to my feet. I watch the wave suck up, dropping out from under me. There is nothing to do but keep going. It's a late take off and really steep. Putting all my weight on my back foot and standing firmly I just make it! The face of the wave races ahead of me and I miss the section. Oh well I'm happy, at least I made the drop.
As I paddle back out to wait for another wave I notice a guy looking at me. I think he is surprised with my wave, probably surprised that I can surf at all. Why is he looking at me so much? I often meet guys out in the water. This time though I'm not sure what it is. I'm feeling something different. I wait for a long time for a wave. Each one that comes there's always someone on it already.
"How you going?" he says with a smile.
"Good thanks. Just trying to get a wave in now," I reply.
Those deep penetrating eyes look deeply into mine as he paddles past. He takes his place back in the line-up not far ahead of me. Soon a wave comes which he paddles for. It looks as though he has the wave so no one else goes for it. He then pulls back and calls to me, "Go, go paddle hard." I paddle as hard as I can and a bit more. I'm determined to get this wave, if only for the fact he has given it to me, and I do.
Over the next few months I continue surfing a few times a week. Ignoring the pain in my body I even start running a little way along the beach back to the car after surfing. I just can't believe it. I can actually do this and I'm

surfing really well! After the past year and a half being so unwell, barely able to even get through each day, it feels so good to be moving and having fun. One day I take my board down to Back Beach. I realise the waves are much bigger than they seemed from the lookout. They are closing out a bit too. I'm reluctant to go out. I watch the big rip that runs alongside the rocks. I know if I jump into it I will be taken out the back easily, so I decide to go. I attach my leg rope and jump into the water. The strong current pulls me along the rip. Only a few paddles and I'm right out the back. There's only one other surfer out here, nicknamed Hairy, and a few more a little way down the beach.

I've only been out the back for a short time and we can see a big set rolling in.

"Here they come. You go this one Di," he urges.

It's a bit daunting but I paddle for the big wave. "You go too, I might not get it," I yell.

We both take off. I jump to my feet, gliding fast behind Hairy along the smooth face of the wave.

"Wooohoooo!" I laugh with exhilaration as we both ride the wave.

Hairy looks behind to see I've made it. He pulls off giving me a free run. I ride along carving up and down the thick shiny face of this powerful wave, faster and faster. In front of me as the wave nears the sand bank I can see it lining up for what looks like a barrel. I've never had a barrel before. Almost twenty years ago I pulled into a wave thinking I might get one. All I got was smashed so I never really tried again. But this looks perfect. I don't know what comes over me. Maybe it's my new-found invincibility. I race along the wave. As the section sucks up I duck down and find myself racing along in a big barrel. Everything happens so fast, but at the same moment time seems to stand still. Nearly all of the hundreds of waves I've caught before I've ridden and moved along the face of the wave. Now in the barrel, I feel like I'm standing still and this amazing powerful green wall of water is sucking upward under my feet. I'm propelling forward through the barrel, surrounded by the wave roaring in my ears. I have no idea what to do. I just stand there and hold on.

I duck down under the lip of the wave a few times and then BANG. Suddenly I hit the water hard. Engulfed and tumbling around in the whitewash I don't know which way is up. Holding my breath I finally come to the surface. Dazed for a moment I realise I'm stinging and tingling all over. I look around. I'm in a thick swarm of small purple jellyfish. Another wave is about to break on top of me. I gasp for a breath as I submerge myself under the wave feeling the soft slimy creatures surrounding me.

Coming to the surface I quickly climb onto my board. I lie there for a moment catching my breath, centring my thoughts. I realise my legs are still being stung so I quickly make my way to the shore.

Standing on the beach looking back out at the waves I'm filled with a combination of exhilaration and fear, joy, pain and excitement. My whole body is buzzing with adrenalin. I'm not sure if it's a positive effect from my big barrel or a negative reaction to the jellyfish. After a short time taking deep relaxing breaths, monitoring what is happening in my body, I come to the conclusion the jellyfish stings have only had a relatively mild effect on me. The initial stinging eases and my heart rate calms. Amazed at what I've just experienced I stand in awe looking out at the ocean. I watch Hairy catch a wave almost all the way in and walk up the beach.

"That was a ripper that wave you got." he exclaims.

"I can't believe it. I got the biggest barrel of my life. And I got the biggest wedgie of my life too!"

I'm on a high for weeks after that wave and of course I share my wonderful achievement with anyone who is happy to listen. I realise that the waves themselves have pushed me to achieve much more than I thought I could. The ocean is alive and once you enter her world you're at her mercy. She has shown me I am much stronger than I realised, or maybe she has made me that way. I now find myself in the contradictory situation of feeling so strong and powerful but at the same time still so sick as the agony within persists.

Beneath the surface of things I am terrified. Terrified because this pain in my body and the reactions I have after eating continue to make me feel awful every day. Though I'm glad I'm so much better, I'm terrified I will never get fully well. I hate feeling this way. Between being a Mum, surfing, and studying hard I'm keeping very busy. Whenever I'm not busy I feel terrible, and it's still very difficult to get a good night's sleep. My anxiety levels are so high but I'm certain it's not just anxiety. It's been over six months since having my tooth out which has helped me to regain a lot of my health, but it doesn't explain these relentless reactions after eating. I can't bear the thought of spending the rest of my life feeling this way. Something *must* be causing it. I know how much breathwork has helped me before and I have experienced the strange 'coincidences' that seem to happen so I set more intentions.

With determination I say to myself over and over, "I intend to get to the bottom of my health problems. I intend to get to the bottom of my health problems. I intend to be one hundred percent healthy." I repeat this regularly as I take deep, relaxed breaths into my belly. Within a week I find myself reading a book called *The Cure for All Diseases,* by Dr Hulda Clark. To my surprise it's filled with very interesting information. The more I read the more intrigued I become. Most of the treatments in this book are the same or similar to those which have helped me so far.

There's the dental clean up, parasite cleanse, kidney cleanse, liver cleanse and liver flush. The liver flush is a lot more intense than the liver cleanses I've done. I know I couldn't have done it when I was extremely unwell, but now without a doubt, I know I need to give it a go. Dr Clark says we all have stones in our liver, even up to two thousand of them, and removing these stones can be one of the best things anyone can do for their health.

I get all the ingredients for the flush and become very nervous. What if nothing happens? What will I do then? I'll still have no answers and nowhere else to turn. It's amazing how hope can keep you going, but on the flip side when you run out of answers and run out of hope it can crush you.

I prepare the ingredients for the liver cleanse. It's a twenty-four-hour procedure and quite intense. I stop eating at 2 pm. At 6 pm I have my first dose of Epsom salts. Around this time a few arguments are brewing in our house and there are demands for my attention. I'm quite annoyed about this. I'm taking time to look after myself, my time for healing. I shouldn't have to be dealing with these silly problems. Despite my attempts to diffuse the situation so I can concentrate on myself and this cleansing process, the tension escalates. I find myself becoming angry and frustrated. In fact anger begins to boil up within me. I know I have to take responsibility for my own feelings and reactions so I remove myself from the tense situation, focus my thoughts, and pay attention to how I am feeling.

Suddenly another wave of negative thoughts and feelings is erupting. Thoughts and feelings that I have suppressed and held within myself for a long time are boiling over. I realise that by trying to keep the peace in many life situations I'm actually holding in a lot of resentment and not acknowledging the reality of many situations. I begin to accept how annoyed or angry I'm feeling, instead of telling myself it's okay when actually it's not. It feels such a relief to allow myself to do this. Suddenly the anger I was feeling disappears and I feel very happy and relieved.

I think about Louise Hay's book *You Can Heal Your Life* which I have studied many times in the past. Again I'm amazed at the emotional connections to physical illnesses. Problems relating to the liver are well known to be related to anger, bitterness and resentment. I think about the tick bites being related to irritation, anger and annoyance, and I can see how I was trying to ignore these feelings and what was creating them. I realise that for so long I've been trying to make myself not have these feelings and to keep the peace with everyone in my life. But in doing so those feelings have become more and more deep seated in my body. I am beginning to see it is in the process of allowing myself to feel these feelings, to acknowledge just how angry and hurt I have felt that I can release those feelings and the energy blockages they cause.

8 pm and it's time for my second lot of Epsom salts. It isn't too hard to get this dose down, unlike the 10 pm concoction that follows - a mixture of olive oil and grapefruit juice. This is disgusting I think to myself. But I don't care. I need to give it a try.

I gulp the mixture down as quickly as I can. Then following the instructions, I lie down and go to bed immediately. Apparently I might feel the stones moving along the bile ducts. Sure enough I do, just under my ribs on the right hand side. It's really weird.

In the morning I feel nauseous. Argh I hate feeling this way. The flush takes effect and with a couple of trips to the toilet I feel fine again. I take the third dose of Epsom salts followed two hours later by the fourth and final dose. While hopeful of some sort of result I'm fearful nothing will happen and I'll be back to the drawing board. Thankfully my fears are short lived. The whole process happens exactly as described in the book. By the following morning I have a collection of sixty-three stones. I'm dumbfounded by the sheer size and number of them. This is just amazing. I don't notice any improvement until my body has settled down over a few days. Again no dramatic improvement but I definitely notice some easing of the reactions after eating.

Hoping my condition will continue to improve I look forward to the second cleanse in a fortnight. I'm so relieved when I have similar results. Again I feel the stones moving. This time the area around my liver is a little more tender. Not quite painful. Just like a small stitch. No wonder. The stones look like a handful of gravel. Some of them sharp and pointy! This is just phenomenal. I can't believe it. I continue with the liver cleanses every fortnight as recommended in the book and my health continues to improve. I photograph and document every single stone for evidence that something was not right in my body.

Coincidently I come across Dr Sandra Cabot's liver cleansing book and remember seeing her years ago on television, speaking about the importance of liver cleansing. I have great admiration for these doctors who step out and use these methods that are not widely practised. I wonder how our society's health would be different now if these principles were adopted by mainstream.

While my health is slowly progressing I'm a little worried about Lily. She often has symptoms of a cold and a few digestive upsets. In fact she has done so for a long time now. Having some dyslexia, and finding it very hard to concentrate and remember things, she is also having difficulties with her schoolwork, which she previously had no problem with. At dancing her teacher always has to repeat the instructions and push her more than the other girls. I have Lily tested for parasites. The doctor says there is no problem and everything is fine. I'm a little dismayed wondering what else it could be. At the counter on leaving I ask for the results. I'm surprised to see she has in fact tested positive for the exact parasite I was having her tested for. The pathology report says 'no action required'. 'Does this give the doctor reason to tell me all is fine?' I wonder. Claire warns me that her son had the same parasite which got into his liver and made him very unwell. I try a number of different parasite remedies but she does not seem to improve.

In a few weeks Lily passes out unexpectedly. Over the next week she has strange spells where everything goes a bit blurry and she feels like she is in a dream. Sometimes she sees stars and feels like she might pass out again. Worried, I take her to a different doctor. He advises it might be wise to have a brain scan. I consider this but fill with dread at the idea. In hope I turn to Dr Clark's *Cure For All Diseases* and read the section on seizures. She says they are often caused by ascaris larvae in the brain. I wonder if this can be true? I read her warning that ascaris eggs are present everywhere in animal filth. Dogs, cats, horses and pigs. I think of all the animals Lily has been around all her life.

Dr Clark's method of treating parasites uses a herbal remedy combined with the use of one of her inventions called the 'zapper'. In her early work Dr Clark monitored the frequency of parasites, viruses and bacteria and could test for that frequency to see if someone has a specific parasite. She discovered that by giving that frequency to the person the pathogen would be killed. During her experimentation using a battery operated device she discovered that any positively offset frequency, anything from 10Hz to 500,000 Hz with sufficient voltage of 5-10 volts, worked to kill most pathogens. And so, the zapper was created. Dr Clark has all of her recipes and instructions for the zapper in her book, which shows me clearly that she's very passionate about sharing all of her information for the health and benefit of everyone, not just as a money-making tool. There is also a modern computerised version of the zapper available.

Danni's husband being an air-conditioning mechanic is very happy to make one for me. For just twenty dollars my zapper is complete. Danni already reports success after trying it out on herself. After one day of feeling very unwell, apparently due to the 'die off' of parasites, she's feeling incredibly good. In fact, better than she's done for many years she tells me.
Lily begins her treatment holding the two copper pipes, one in each hand. We follow the instructions. Three zaps of seven minutes with a twenty-minute gap in between. I'm cautious because Dr Clark warns to go slowly at first because the zapping can actually trigger seizures but they will quickly end when the parasites are killed. Despite my concern I know this is something we need to try. With the full treatment complete Lily feels no side effects. Nor does she have any over the next few days. The next week she notices some big changes.
"Have you been doing lots of practise Lily?" asks Rebecca, her dance teacher.
"Umm, mmm," Lily gives half a nod.
"You're doing really well!"
Suddenly able to concentrate and remember a lot more, Lily's school work also improves dramatically. A number of months later I see the teacher who takes her special maths class.
"You know, for the first few months Lily wasn't retaining any information. I kept saying to her, 'concentrate Lily, we have done this,' and we would go over and over the same things, her teacher recalls. "Then suddenly she just started getting it and has taken off ever since."
I'm amazed and elated. I knew Lily had gone from the special maths class to topping her normal maths class, but I hadn't realised there was such a sudden improvement in her work exactly at that time when we did the zapping. The teacher is wide eyed and enthralled as I explain about the electrical contraption I've used to treat Lily.
It has now been six months since Dad passed away and I receive fines of hundreds of dollars for a few road tolls worth a few dollars that I forgot to pay during my visits to see him. When I call the relevant number to discuss the situation I'm given another number to call. The lady nicely tells me that I have to call the department I have just spoken to. I call them back and they quite definitely tell me I must call the other number. I feel myself becoming extremely agitated. After about six or seven phone calls, I finally speak to someone who seems to know what they are talking about. As I explain that I used that road on my way to visit my dying

father, I see the road in my mind. I feel my throat closing up. I am trying to get the words out but I can barely breathe now.

"It's okay love, I know what you are going through," the lady on the phone comforts me.

"I'm … sorry. Just … a … minute." I put the phone down and try to pull myself together. I don't want to go through another fifty phone calls to sort this out. I take a few deep breaths and pick up the phone again.

"I'm … sorry …I'd … really like … to … get this … sorted."

I feel like an elastic band is around the inside of my throat choking me. I cannot hold back my grief. I feel very embarrassed but the lady on the phone is so lovely. By the end of the call we have everything sorted out and I feel like I have just spoken to Lifeline. I cry and cry for my father and eventually I feel a huge relief. I guess that was bound to happen sometime.

Over the next eight months I begrudgingly carry out the liver flush every two, three or four weeks. Despite my aversion to the process, the results are well worth it. So far I've removed around six hundred stones, many of them pea-sized. Some larger than a five-cent piece. Though I still struggle with each cleanse I notice improvements. My reactions after eating, the buzzing, aching and cramping in my muscles all ease noticeably, as do the heart palpitations. My whole body becomes more relaxed. I dread going to sleep because I still wake every morning feeling awful and experience agony every day, but I begin to sleep through most of the night and thank goodness, I get some decent blissful sleep.

I'm surfing all the time now, every day in fact. It's amazing to be able to keep on going day after day. I haven't been able to do this in over fifteen years. I'm not too sure if it's a good thing though. I know I'm living on adrenalin all the time. I wish I could stop it surging through my body, but it's nonstop all day every day, so I just go with it. Out surfing I know when my body has had enough. I often hit a point where I feel a strange collapse in the strength in my back with very jittery weak feelings.

Day by day I try to listen to my body and rest if I'm tired, but when resting I don't feel rested, and despite my improvements the agitation in my body continues to scream at me, making it more comfortable to just keep going. I know people talk to me and see me looking so fit and strong, but they have no idea the agony within that I hide.

I often wonder if I'm pushing myself too much but I have plenty of energy and I'm having so much fun that I don't want to stop. I don't want to stop and rest and feel the agony in my body if I can be sitting in the ocean feeling relief from that agony. I can't help but check the surf every morning and get out there each day no matter what the conditions.

One afternoon I see Mr Dark Eyes, the one who gave me that wave during my first surf out the point. Beer in hand he is talking to the boys. I don't know why I feel so drawn to him.

"What was I thinking?" I ask myself. "Maybe I was imagining things?"

He's not bad looking, but he's elusive and outspoken. That may have suited me in the past, but not now.

Following a few months of small surf over winter a big swell comes up out of the blue. Everyone is keen for a wave. On the beach I see Dave 'Baddy' Treloar, our local legendary surfer and long-time resident of Angourie, who starred in the iconic 70's surf film *Morning of the Earth*.

"I'll follow you and I should be right hey Baddy?" I exclaim with a laugh.

He gives me a big grin as I paddle out behind him. He sits on his own on the big dumpy beach break while I keep paddling out to the softer wave at Angourie Back Point, joining a long line of surfers. Every now and then I notice a really big set breaking way out. Though it's absolutely huge it looks perfect, peeling off left and right. I don't understand why all these guys aren't over there. I can't believe no one is there. It looks beautiful. If I were a strong, fit young guy I'd go over there.

Another big set pulses through breaking left and right. Watching the big peaks peeling along launching into barrelly sections, I know that people travel the world looking for waves like this. The picture in front of me could easily be in the pages of a surfing magazine. An excited wave of adrenalin rushes through my body. Bugger it. I *am* going over there. It isn't too far to paddle from the point but from the beach it's at least a couple of hundred metres or more. It feels like I'm way out in the ocean on my own. Hang on I *am* way out in the ocean on my own. Looking down into the deep dark water below I ignore the unease that creeps through my body, reassuring myself all is fine.

I'm a bit nervous. I don't really know if I'll even have the courage to catch one of these waves. In the distance I see a big set rolling in. It's huge. I wonder what on earth I'm doing out here. I'm in the perfect position for the biggest wave of the set. I begin paddling. I'm not really sure if I'll get it. Maybe I will but I'm not sure if I want to get it.

Next thing I hear Baddy screaming at the top of his lungs, "Gooooo, goooo, goooooo!"

I feel myself paddling with all my might. I can see it will probably close out but I go for it anyway. Somehow I find myself taking one of the biggest drops of my life. As I reach to my feet the water drops away under me.

The wave stands up vertically as I torpedo down the steep shiny wall of water. I feel the wind and spray on my face as I career downwards. Hanging on with the tips of my toes, down down I just make the drop as I'm thrust forward. At such a speed a small bump on the water sends me into a big wobble. Holding tight I can hear and feel the power of the enormous wall of water crashing down behind me. Just holding steady I'm racing along trying to keep up with the face of the wave. As it crosses the deeper water of the gutter it fills up a little, now making for easy riding. I glide along the big wide shiny face of the wave just like the seabirds do feeling as free as a bird!
"That was a BOMB!" calls Baddy.
I laugh with a huge smile across my face. I'm sure he is even more surprised than I am. For so many years my health kept me from surfing and I watched the other surfers from the beach with envy. Eventually I became content to just play in the small surf with the kids. Many people probably didn't even know that I could surf and now, here I am catching the 'Bombs'. I'm thrilled to catch one more big wave riding it almost all the way to the beach. I think I have pushed my luck enough for one day and head in.
I am stoked. If Baddy says that was a bomb, I know it was a bomb. I feel like telling the whole world, "Look, look what I have done." Not because I want to show off, but because I'm amazed at the recovery of my physical body. Amazed at the effectiveness of my healing journey. I'm surfing some of the biggest and best waves of my life. Something I had given up on many years ago and never thought I would be doing at over forty years of age. I'm very passionate about healing but I'm even more passionate about moving past healing on to living a healthy and happy life.
On the whole doctors and natural health practitioners are amazing in emergency situations and helping us on the road to recovery when things have gone wrong, but ultimately we have to take responsibility for our own health. I know now that if you really commit, even if it's difficult at times, seemingly insurmountable obstacles can be overcome and amazing things can be achieved.
Sometimes, especially for someone who has been very unwell, those amazing things can simply be a walk in the park or a gathering with friends or family. As long as it inspires you and brings joy to your heart, it is worth it.

10 Portal to Another Dimension

While I'm overjoyed with the strength I've gained and the daily high of surfing, the relentless pain within is a never ending grind of frustration. It feels like it's never ever going to stop. I go over and over what other possible causes there could be for this ill health. Many of my symptoms match Lyme Disease which causes a range of mysterious symptoms and even death, but doctors and health authorities say it's not in Australia. I've had a skin blemish which, for a long time, I thought may have been ring worm. Now as I read more about people whose overseas results have tested positive to Lyme Disease I wonder if this rash was the typical 'bullseye' which often occurs at the site of the tick bite. Either way, whether or not I have Lyme Disease, I've had so much improvement with the treatments I've used I'd prefer to continue on the path I'm on rather than take the high doses of long-term antibiotics used to treat Lyme and risk going backwards.

Every now and then I have sensations of a stitch in my liver. I figure there *must* be more stones. I continue with the liver cleanses, occasionally having little or no stones and only slight improvements. Nonetheless they are improvements and that is something, so I will keep at it until I'm sure they're all gone. Day after day I consider the possibility that anxiety is causing these horrendous symptoms, but it just doesn't add up. Despite my diagnosis I'm sure as ever that my condition has not been purely that. I've had so much anxiety in the past and these physical symptoms are different. Twelve years ago after the ordeal in Tasmania I would have happily accepted such a diagnosis. No doubt I was affected by Post Traumatic Stress Disorder for quite some time and while there were very good reasons for my severe anxiety, I certainly never had the plethora of physical symptoms that I have now.

Back then Jemma was eight months old. I talked Mike into a move back to his island home, to the beautiful property he had bought many years ago. Over traffic lights and suburbia, I didn't want to be pushing a pram through the streets. I wanted to put on a sling and be walking through the bush or sitting out in the paddock with the horses, growing our own food and living a self-sufficient lifestyle. With the horses loaded into a truck and most of our belongings in a removalist van we were on our way. A cool and icy breeze on our faces, we watch the sun rise from the horizon as the ferry nears Tasmania. Following the winding roads through the beautiful countryside we arrive at the small town where Mike grew up.

His parents are very happy to see us. Thrilled to spend time with their granddaughter. Over the following weeks Mike, his father and two brothers Greg and Sam, work hard cutting logs to create our new home. Some old iron from the family farm takes its place on the roof and our new home, this beautiful little log cabin looking as if it has been here for years, is now complete. We don't have power or running water. Well, actually we do have running water. It's running past in the creek nearby. We're very happy with the drum heater which Greg has made for us to cook and boil water on. Our only source of power, it gives off a huge amount of warmth fulfilling our heating needs.

"How many other women do you know who have a candlelit dinner every night?" Mike exclaims proudly with a grin.

The air is so cold we barely need refrigeration, but we're heading towards summer so buying a large roll of hessian Mike constructs a Cool Gardy safe. It doesn't take long and we're settled in nicely. Sitting on the veranda we're surrounded by bush. Fairy wrens fluttering among the mossy growths join the symphony of birds enjoying their morning chorus. Wallabies nibble grass around the base of the ferns, as the sound of water trickling along the rocks and waterfalls in the creek bed fills the air. Having strolled down the hill the horses sniff and nudge us over the veranda eager for their morning treat.

Wandering down along the creek bed we fill our mouths with luscious fresh blackberries. Jemma squashes them in her hands, dark juices running down her arms. We watch the big black fresh water lobsters slowly moving around in the water. As we come to the river we see platypus swimming along the surface. They disappear under the water, only to pop up a little way downstream. While our river block is flat the rest of the property is a steep hill. With Jemma in a carrier on Mike's back we climb to the top along tracks through the bush, past wombat holes and the natural springs, which give the horses a continual supply of water. Eventually we reach the top of the hill. With a 360-degree view the outlook is magnificent. The river meanders its way through the valley surrounded by mountain ranges as far as the eye can see.

Walking down the other side of the hill we drop in to visit Mrs Flynn. In her eighties she is now on her own after her husband passed away a few years ago. They had a rule there would be no whiskey before 11 am. A rule Mrs Flynn always keeps! We sit and chat until eventually strolling home along the dirt road. It's so peaceful here. No traffic or neighbours close by. Just the sounds of the bush and all the creatures within. I often just stand. Looking around at all the plants and animals I soak up the glorious energy which nature so generously offers.

Most afternoons Mike brings home fresh fish for tea. Today Greg is teaching him how to fly fish. Quietly standing knee deep in waterproof fishing pants Mike and Greg throw their lines, alternating between the rapids and the calmer deep waters.

"I'm heading home," Mike says.

"If you wait a minute I'll give you a ride," Greg offers.

"No, I'll just walk along the river."

"The owner of that property there won't like it," Greg warns.

"What do you mean? No one owns the river. He can't stop me walking home along the riverbank."

Fishing rod over his shoulder Mike wanders towards home. The sky turns grey as the last rays of sun fade. The air becomes cool and a soft mist rises above the water. The techniques that his brother has been teaching him fill Mike's thoughts. He startles at the sound of snapping twigs in the bushes ahead. He stops. Standing quietly, he looks around. 'Must be roos,' he thinks to himself and continues along the river's edge.

Suddenly a man jumps out waving a gun, screaming hysterically, "Get off, what are you doing?"

"I'm just walking home!" Mike yells holding his arms out.

"Get off my land! You. What are you doing here? What are you doing! Get off!"

Mike stumbles backwards, retreating as quickly as he can. "I'm just walking home along the river," he tries to explain. The man continues screaming and waving the gun in Mike's face. Mike can barely understand what he's saying.

Mike finally reaches the side boundary. He joins his brother and the other fishermen who have come to see what's going on.

"You alright?" asks Greg.

"Yeah, I'm ok," says Mike shakily.

"You bloody idiot. I told you he was a nutter! That was that bloody Albert Naylor."

After stoking up the fire to get the water boiling the rice is almost cooked. I hear noise outside. "How did you go?" I call.

No response. The dogs seem unsettled. I open the door and they run out onto the veranda. Back to my cooking I stir the rice adding some herbs and seasoning.

"Stop that barking," I call to the dogs.

"Where's that Daddy, Jem?" I pick her up and go outside. Hearing footsteps I look into the darkness.
"How'd you go?"
"Got some dinner," Mike replies holding up a big trout, looking visibly shaken.
"What's the matter?"
"The bloody neighbour down the river jumped out waving a gun at me."
He explains everything as we both sit in shock.
The next day we talk with Greg about whether or not to go to the police. We choose not to for fear of aggravating the situation. Two days later Greg arrives looking very upset. Albert has accused him of threatening to kill him so the police, against their will, have had to charge Greg. Mike enquires whether Albert mistook Greg for himself. The police say he insists it was Greg. After listening to all the statements they charge Albert with aggravated assault with a deadly weapon.
The police tell us the 'big fellas' have drug raided him twice but somehow he always comes up clean. I'm shocked to learn of the extent of the troubles Albert has given so many people. It's almost a week since the incident. With our food stock getting low it's time for some shopping. Mike and I put the dogs in the shed and head into town. On our return the dogs are gone. I call them in panic.
"Do you think he's got them," I ask Mike tearfully.
Searching everywhere we can't find them. I walk down the driveway and onto the road. Looking over towards Albert's house I scour his land. As I glance over the fields everything becomes a blur, dreamlike. Mike decides to ring the dog pound on the slight chance they may have them. To our surprise and relief they do. As it turns out Albert rang the police to ask about his rights to shoot dogs on his property so the sergeant came straight out to pick them up. We're not sure how the dogs got out. The main thing is we have them back.
Standing looking out over that paddock, terrified that our beloved dogs may have been shot, thinking how close Mike was to losing his life, I went into some form of shock. Somehow another dimension opened. My spirit, my soul, went somewhere ... somewhere I had not been for many, many years. I didn't know it at the time, but I was about to embark on a journey. A very deep, dark and mystical journey.

Di Ellis

11 Drawn into a Primal, Dark and Magical World

Although my serene paradise has been shattered I try my hardest not to let it get to me. It's Saturday night and we find our way to a party. Warmly welcomed and introduced to many locals we join in the vibrant dancing and drumming. When asked where I live I'm told about the mad man who lives down there. One lady rubs her fingers together and tells me about dealings of 'the white stuff'. The guy next to her tells stories about the arsenal of guns hidden beneath a concrete slab and the machine gun used to mow kangaroos in half. I feel the blood drain from my face.
"That's just what I want to hear," I state.
He apologises profusely realising it isn't an appropriate party story. Learning to block these things out of my mind I chat and mingle enjoying the rest of the evening as best I can.
Summer is drawing near, bringing some very warm days. We enjoy swimming in the icy-cold water hole, exploring the countryside and getting to know the community. We often visit Mike's family or they come to see us. It's nice watching Jemma get to know her grandparents. She's always straight up to Pop's strawberry patch.
Just up the road is a beautiful little Welsh Mountain pony. They tell me he's a wild stallion who's never been handled. A horse trainer apparently tried to catch him once but he broke through the yard and they didn't bother again. The property was recently sold and the new owners have just moved in. Word has it they don't want this wild pony.
"Perfect," I think. I'm unable to catch him but he's happy to follow Molly as I ride her home. I admire his beautiful thick long main and forelock. "I'm going to call you Wizard" I spend many hours sitting on the ground throwing out bits of bread, coaxing him closer. Sometimes if I move a little he bolts away in fright. Over time though his trust builds until eventually he's happy to come and sniff and nuzzle my head. I'm filled with joy as my relationship with this gorgeous pure soul deepens.
Albert tries all he can to make our lives uncomfortable with continuous spurious complaints of harassment, accusing us of discrimination towards his Asian wife, washing nappies in the creek, boundary disputes and more. Officials from council, government departments and the police are at our doorstep weekly profusely apologising that they have to respond to all complaints but have no intention of following anything up.
Knowing Mrs Flynn has received the same neighbourly response over the years we pay her a visit. Puffing away on her cigarette she talks of the

harassment she and her deceased husband received over the years. Their dogs were shot, dead possums in the water tank, gunshots fired over their heads and more. Twenty years ago Mrs Flynn lost her son in a motor bike accident. Every year since then his motorcycle gang come and stay with her, cutting and chopping enough wood to last her the winter. She and her husband tried to keep the trouble quiet but the gang got word of it. They never had any more trouble after that. Mike would like to go and 'sort the bastard out' but I'm terrified of what could happen.

I attend a workshop with my meditation group, called 'Analysing Your Dreams'. I find the information and techniques surprisingly effective and feel an immediate affinity for Diane the counsellor who runs the workshops. Feeling the stress from recent events I make an appointment for Mike and I to see Diane for a counselling session. It's a relief to talk about all we've been through. Since the troubles with Albert I feel like a fog has come over me. A very dark fog. Many feelings of grief have been triggered. Simple things that I would normally handle easily now seem difficult. I know this huge amount of grief I feel is related to my childhood so I continue to see Diane every fortnight.

"So tell me about your family?" she asks.

I've learnt how to tell this story in an entertaining way that people can almost follow. "Well, I was adopted at birth. My adopted parents were nearly fifty and they had two of their own children, who were around twenty. I also had a sister a couple of years older who was adopted. When I was three and a half my adopted mother died. When I was five Dad remarried. My step mother also adopted me and she had four of her own children."

"Right, I think I've got that,' says Diane. "Now, can you repeat what you said about your adopted mother but this time say it without laughing?"

As I continue my throat closes, so much so I can barely breathe. Slowly my grief begins to overflow. With Diane's support I release grief I have suppressed for many years. I feel a huge relief. She explains the laughing is a defence mechanism people often use to keep them from feeling the pain. I see Diane fortnightly for quite a while until I reach a point where I feel like I need something more.

"I feel like I need something deeper, like there's all this stuff inside. But I can't get to it or release it,' I confess. I ask Diane if she knows anyone who does rebirthing and she gives me the number of a lady called Anne, who does breath and body work.

I have no idea of the incredible journey ahead. Not a journey by land or air but a journey through time and creation to my soul within. This journey has certainly not been instigated by choice but through necessity to cope. In the years to come I will realise the importance of the incredible understanding and wisdom I'm about to develop. It will hold me strongly, steadfastly through the greatest challenges to my physical, mental and emotional health, giving me strength to stand strong in the face of ignorance and corruption, but most of all, it will hold me through the darkest fears and doubts held deep within myself which ultimately have created it all.

I call Anne and make an appointment. With her warm and open embrace I feel immediately comfortable. "Now this is quite different to counselling," she explains, guiding me through to a room where I lie down on a mattress. Having turned on some relaxing music, she sits on a cushion next to me and talks me through a few relaxation exercises.

"Feel yourself sinking deeply into the mattress. Your whole body relaxed. Notice any sensations or feelings in your body. Nice full relaxed breaths into your belly. Letting go of any thoughts pay attention to your breathing and your body sensations. Allow yourself to feel how your body feels."

I am lying there for quite some time.

"So what's happening in your belly?"

"Um, it just feels really tense, like a rock." I don't know how she knew something was happening in my belly as I have a blanket over me and haven't moved.

"That's fine. Allow yourself to feel that feeling. It will probably move or change."

"It just feels stuck there," I report.

"Allow yourself to feel those stuck feelings. Remember to breathe."

I realise I'm holding my breath. "I'm feeling very angry."

Anne assures me it's alright to be angry. But I don't want to be angry. I want to be happy and peaceful. Anne explains that often those angry feelings will change into a different feeling. Five or ten minutes pass and I'm still stuck in the angry feeling. Anne wants to know if there's any reason why I can't allow myself to feel angry? I don't say anything. My breathing becomes very rapid. An image appears in my mind. I can see my adopted mother in the hospital. I just want to hit her and scream at her to get up.

"Because I am not supposed to. And it would upset everyone else even more."

"And how is your belly feeling now?" Anne asks.

"Churning and angry."

She suggests I yell if I want to. But I figure there's no point. Anne encourages me to give this a try and see what happens, assuring me I can stop any time."
I lie still. I am frozen.
"Take a breath Di," she prompts.
I realise I'm holding my breath again.
"Nice full relaxed breaths. What would you say if you could?"
"Get up."
"Ok, good. You can say anything you want to say. Nothing will surprise me. You can scream into the pillows if you want to."
At first I say it softly. Gradually I begin yelling until I hear myself screaming," Get up. Get up, I hate you. What are you doing?"
"You can hit the pillows if you want to."
I am now screaming hysterically, hitting and punching pillows, slamming them down on the mattress, over and over. Eventually my anger turns into deep grief. A feeling that takes over my whole body. It seems like it will never go away. I curl up into a ball on the mattress crying, while Anne rubs my back.
I lie there not moving for quite some time. Slowly I begin to notice that the churning feelings in my belly are completely gone. I feel such a relief. This is strange. My belly is feeling really nice. Soon a deep hearty laugh spontaneously rises from within me. I look at Anne who is smiling at me warmly.
"I feel so happy. This is so strange. Why do I feel so happy?"
"Laughing is a good sign that you've had a big release."
At the end of my session I make another appointment to see Anne.
"Now be gentle on yourself. You might feel a little different for a while."
I look forward to seeing Anne every fortnight, each session unlocking another layer of 'stuck' energy in my body. Taking me to a deeper level of love and understanding of myself. Though I still have feelings of grief, I'm beginning to feel a wonderful deep peace and love I've never felt before. We work with whatever arises during the session. Images and memories, feelings and sensations in my body. Anne never pushes me in any direction in particular. Nor does she suggest anything. She just guides and encourages me to listen to my body. To accept myself and my feelings. I'm experiencing a whole new side to myself that I've never known before.
One session I hear myself begin to make a wailing sound on each breath out. Gradually it builds stronger and louder, becoming an enormous deep crying out moan. It's very strange. I don't feel sad at all. It just feels like

something my body needs to do. As it's happening I'm thinking about a movie I watched years ago. The main character had been in a bad accident and was hospitalised. She was doing this exact same moaning. I could barely stand to watch it. I thought how ridiculous it was. I knew that no one would actually do that. Well, I thought I knew. This deep primal moan goes on for a very long time until a beautiful, calm peacefulness sweeps over my body. I bathe in this heavenly sensation. Eventually I open my eyes. Anne is smiling at me one hand holding mine, the other on my shoulder. I don't need to say anything. She knows that I'm amazed by this experience. I know that she knows it's perfectly normal.

I'm astounded by some of the thoughts, feelings and memories I'm having. A number of years ago one of my aunts told me that her daughter had done rebirthing. My cousin remembered things that happened when she was in the womb and asked my aunt whether they were correct. To her surprise, they were. Although my aunt is very honest, down-to-earth and 'straight laced' I found this very difficult to believe. How could you possibly remember something that happened when you were in the womb? Now though I'm beginning to have thoughts, visions and dreams, which are inexplicable. One morning I awake from a dream in which my grandfather was a policeman. He drove to a house looking for my mother who was pregnant with me. She was having fun with her friends riding a mattress down the stairs. He was very angry at her and a big fight erupted. I don't know what this dream means, but somehow it seems relevant. I notice a definite pattern of events that are happening in my life. I begin to write down the time frames when particular events occurred. I also notice a correlating pattern of events during both of my pregnancies.

During one of my sessions I have a strong feeling of being in the womb. I can sense everything that is happening around my mother. Particularly how everyone is feeling. There is so much fighting and misery. I know I do not want to be there.

"Can I possibly be remembering things that happened when I was in the womb?" I ask Anne in disbelief.

"Yep, you sure can." she replies. "It's actually very common and quite simple when you think about it. We have a body memory, or cellular memory, which holds feelings and memories all of our lives. Just like riding a bike. You may not have ridden a bike for years but your body remembers how to do it. That's why now you're a mother you've had so many of these feelings around your mothers."

"That makes so much sense. And it makes me feel so much better knowing where all these feelings are coming from, instead of just being really confused about them."
"That's right. But it's not just what's in the past. It's the patterns we are in now, that were created by our past experiences."
"Yeah. I think I'm getting it. It still feels a bit weird. But it's a good weird."
Trying to piece together all my visions, images, feelings and dreams is like trying to complete a jigsaw with pieces from a number of different jigsaws. But somehow they fit together. The more they fit together the more the story that I have been told about who my birth father is falls apart, and with that comes more confusion. The thoughts and feelings I'm having completely contradict what I've been told. I can't bear it.
I make some phone calls explaining that I'm feeling really confused. I would like to know what happened when I was in the womb, particularly at around eight weeks, four and a half months, six months and eight months. A car accident? A man was driving. But who? My father, I'm sure. A court case and a big fight! I'm dumbfounded. I make more enquiries and many of the feelings and memories I've had are confirmed. The problem is that even more just doesn't add up.
Ever since becoming a mother I've had a burning desire to meet my father. I've never questioned what I've been told. Now though, I'm having a lot of difficulties. The confusion and grief I'm feeling is affecting my life and my ability to be a good mother. More than anything I do not want to keep repeating the unhealthy patterns that I've been in for most of my life. I will do whatever I can to work out the problems that I feel within myself. I want to be the best mother I can possibly be.
I have very strong feelings about my father. Somehow I can sense what he's like. As if I know him. I need to ring my grandmother. Maybe she can tell me more. As usual we chat for a bit about what we are both growing in our gardens.
"I'm just wondering if you know much about my father Gran? Or anything that may have happened?" I ask.
"I'm afraid I can't tell you much. The only thing I remember is that your grandfather went to check on your mother. She was with some friends and he wanted to see what she was doing."
"And do you know what happened?"
Everything she remembers sounds so similar to my dream! I thank her sincerely. I can't believe it. That's exactly what happened in my dream. Full of curiosity I call my Aunt.
"There was a man,' she tells. 'He was tall like you and he looked like you."

"Really? Do you know his name?"
"I know his first name was Roderick. I'm sorry but I don't remember his last name. He was a radio announcer. You know your mother was planning on keeping you?"
"No I didn't know. She said she was never going to keep me."
"Up until eight months she was. Knitting clothes for you and all, but they talked her into giving you up."
"Who's they?"
"The counsellors or nuns I presume."
"Really? Thank you so much for telling me. You've helped me a lot."
My conscious mind is finding relief from the confusion of unclear and differing stories. Meanwhile though, deep dark emotions that are unlocking from within are taking me to places I have never been before. With Mike working a couple of hours away, we are renting an old house in a little old mining town. With the use of pillows, or a branch on a rock out the back of the house, I have learnt to allow the wild anger from within to release, and release ... and release some more. In fact, I wonder when it will stop releasing. I learn that the previous owner of the house was electrocuted working on the powerlines. I often find myself sitting alone in the centre of a dark room in the middle of the house imagining his energy. I feel his energy. I feel as though I could burn up. From the inside out.
I see Anne for my fortnightly appointment. "It all happened!" I explain excitedly. "All the visions, dreams and memories of the feelings I had from in the womb. They actually happened. And my father. I learnt more about him too."
"Wow," murmurs Anne. "So how are you feeling about it all?"
"Good. Well I can't believe I actually remembered things from in the womb. That's weird. But it makes me feel better in myself, because I don't feel like I'm going crazy. All the mixed up feelings I've been having make sense now. It was real. I don't feel so confused anymore. And my father *was* in the picture. Not that I would tell anyone about that."
"Why not?"
"Because of all the controversy."
"Do you feel ashamed about it?" asks Anne. I say not. "Then why hide it?" she adds.
"I'm upset but I don't want to hurt anyone."
"Why would it hurt anyone?"
I think about this question. I wonder why I feel a need to keep all of this a secret? Why anyone should keep it secret? I feel a strange sense of

confusion. "I'm carrying on the shame aren't I, by hiding it?" I say. "Yes. I'm still carrying the shame by trying to hide it myself. That's it, isn't it?"
"I don't know. That is up to you to determine. It was a long time ago and often when we try to hide things like that there's usually a lot going on behind it. You don't want to be hiding who you are and where you came from. You want to be proud of who you are, no matter what happened. Does that make sense?"
"Absolutely. I felt a wave of excitement just as you said that."
"Well, let's start the session shall we?"
I lie down eagerly as Anne guides me through the relaxation exercises. I look forward to the wonderful feelings I always experience towards the end of a breath session. I feel myself relax deeper and deeper. I don't know how long I've been lying here when I hear Anne's voice, "Take a breath Di."
I realise I'm holding my breath. My whole body is tense. Anne asks how I am, "Like I shouldn't be here," I respond. "Like I should never have been born. Well, no, I don't believe that, but I guess a part of me does. I feel like I need to live through death or something."
"Do you want to die?"
"No!"
"Ok." I sense a slight relief in Anne. "So these feelings you are having, where are they in your body?"
"Everywhere. I feel tense like a rock. Like I can't move."
"Allow those feelings just to be there. Take nice full breaths into your belly."
Feelings that I shouldn't be alive overwhelm me. Overwhelm my whole body. Anne rubs my shoulder reassuringly. Deeper and deeper I go within. My whole body is filled with dread, as I weep.
"What's happening Di?" Anne asks.
"I don't want to be here. I have caused all this trouble and everybody wants to get rid of me. I just want to die."
Anne strokes my arm. "Remember to breathe into your belly, Di."
Gradually the feelings ease. "Now I want you to go within and feel your mother's love for you. This is a deep unconditional love, beyond anything that may be happening in your lives."
I don't see how this will work, but I give it a try. "I don't feel anything."
"That's okay. Though you can't feel it at the moment know there is a deep love from your mother that is unconditional. It can never be taken away. It's a part of who you are."

Again I focus deep within. I lie here for a long time with different feelings and sensations running through my body. To my surprise a feeling of incredibly deep love and joy begins to fill me. I can do nothing but smile. Soon Anne encourages me to go through the same process with my father. Strongly sensing his energy, his soul, again I am filled with profound feelings of deep love. My tears now are tears of joy. Deep feelings of love and wholeness fill my body, unlike anything I have ever felt before. It is truly wonderful. Eventually I open my eyes to Anne's smiling face. "That was amazing!" I exclaim.
"Now those feelings are yours," Anne points out. "A part of you to hold within. Always."
I am amazed at the incredible depth of love I'm able to connect with from the past. Or maybe it's not from the past but rather from spirit, which is timeless. This connection goes deeper than personality. Deeper than any event or trauma that may have occurred. Deeper than the physical body. It's totally pure and life-giving. I see that no matter what trauma you may have lived through, no matter how bad a relationship may be with your loved ones, this soul love which we all have at our core for each other, is so very much deeper than any of that, and is vitally important to all of us.
I see Anne regularly and know to the depths of my soul, my spirit is safe as I develop a profound trust in her. I'm realising just how important it is for anyone who has had any form of abandonment, rejection, or trust issues to have this type of faith in a practitioner. In fact I am learning how important it is for everyone to have someone in their life who they trust with their deepest vulnerabilities. Any slight feeling of mistrust creates an environment of shutting down and closing off, not only emotionally but also physically. Therefore having someone whose company you feel safe in, to express your deepest self, is incredibly expanding and healing.
It's almost been one year since I first saw Anne. I don't know if I've ever felt so open and free to allow my true self to slowly but surely emerge. To my great fortune, Anne is not only a breath and bodywork practitioner, but also a homebirth midwife as I am now expecting another baby. Once again I relish having a baby growing inside me. My appointments combine check-ups to take all the necessary observations. Just as Claire said, the true role of the midwife is not to birth the baby, but to keep the mother protected from outside influences, so the mother is safe to birth the baby in her own way and time, unhindered. This is also how I feel during my sessions with Anne. She allows me to feel safe so I am able to feel and express whatever emotions or feelings are within.

Quantum Health

Once again, early in my pregnancy I have a threatened miscarriage. This time though I feel very differently about the threat of losing this baby. I desperately want to keep the baby, but I am tired. I have a two year old to care for and life is just harder. I want to cry. I want to be scared. I am scared, but this time I surrender to the universe. I say to myself, "If it is meant to be, it will be."

We're also preparing for two foals. My horses Molly and Lola have become extremely round. I calculate the probable due date for the foals. As May approaches I check the mares many times a day. With huge bellies their udders are filling with milk. It's not long before Lola has a beautiful baby boy we call Zulu. One week later Molly has a little girl who we name Zara. As they grow they begin to play and chase each other around the paddock, always making sure not to go too far from their mums.

Although Albert was ordered to hand over his guns, every now and then we hear a shot go off in the middle of the night. We have become a little used to it, but it still keeps us on edge. With a growing belly I'm beginning to wake in the night more often. This is quite a nuisance when you have an outhouse. Quietly I hop up trying not to wake Mike and Jemma. With a small torch I make my way down the veranda stairs and along the track by the side of the cabin. The moon shines through the trees nearby casting a shadow along the ground. With no streetlights for miles, I admire the stars shining so brightly. Stepping carefully through the dark I return back to the cabin. I open the door and begin to step inside. Suddenly the door is thrown back on to me with Mike yelling behind it.

"It's me, it's me," I scream.

Mike grabs me, holding me tight. "Shit, I thought it was Albert coming in. I'm sorry. I'm sorry. Are you alright?"

"Yeah I'm ok," I reassure him. 'Just hurt my hand a bit, but it's okay."

A few weeks later it's a beautiful clear day and I'm having a quiet ride on Cobba. It crosses my mind to be careful riding while I'm pregnant but I have one hundred percent faith in my old boy. We know each other so well. We wander the tracks through the bush and along the top of the ridge. Making our way back down we criss-cross the steep hill. From up here I can see Albert in his fruit orchard, his bright orange hair glowing in the sun. I feel jittery. I'm nervous just seeing him. But I won't let him think he has got the better of me. His dogs up in the house yard start barking a warning. Albert must be expecting Mike to ride past on his pushbike as he often does. I watch him as he crouches, hiding behind a bush, trying to see what the dogs are barking at. Little does he know I'm behind him watching everything he's doing.

Di Ellis

I cannot help myself. "Yooohooooo," I call.
Startled, he jumps up, looks around to see me waving, then pretends to be doing something. I continue on with my ride with a sense of defiant satisfaction.
"I won't let you get the better of me you bastard," I think to myself.

12 Surrender

With my baby now due in three weeks I see Anne weekly for check-ups.
"I still feel like there's unresolved 'stuff' inside," I tell her. "I really wanted to have it all dealt with by now so when I have this baby everything would be as good as it could be."
"It will be as good as it can be,' she assures me. 'It will be just as it's meant to be." Somehow Anne knows just what to say when I need it. There are a couple of dates she won't be available. Although I wasn't planning to have a backup midwife, I'm getting a bit nervous so I meet with another lovely midwife who is available if need be.
Around my due date I have a call from Errol. He informs me that dad has just been in for a triple heart bypass operation and is doing okay. He didn't want to worry me so never even mentioned it. I try to calm myself as much as I can. I am shocked, but relieved he is doing well. Typical dad, not saying anything about it so not to worry me.
A few days later I have a phone call from the police sergeant. "Hi Dianne. Sorry to bother you. Albert has called saying your horses are out on the road?"
I look out the window. "I can't see them just now. I'll go down and have a look." Jemma and I walk down our long driveway to the bottom gate. Sure enough the horses are on the road. Opening the gate I rattle a bucket with some feed in it. Eagerly, the horses come over. "What do you lot think you're doing? You'll get me in trouble.," I say closing the gate behind them, careful to keep my big belly out of harm's way.
I am now a week overdue and no baby in sight. I go out to feed the horses. Lola and Zulu are not in sight either. "That's strange," I call to Mike. "Where's Lola and Zulu?" My heart is beating very fast. I know something is wrong. It is not like Lola to stay away from the other horses. Molly maybe, but not Lola. "Mike, there's something wrong." I walk along the track, looking into the bushes as far as I can see. "Lola. Zulu," I call and whistle over and over.
I'm relieved to finally see Lola coming through the bushes. But Zulu is not with her.
Lola is very distressed. "Come here girl." I rub her neck, trying to comfort her. I want to tell her it's okay but I don't think it is.
Mike puts his arm around me. "Take it easy. I've just called Greg. He's coming over. We'll go search up the hill." A few minutes later they head up the hill. It's not long before they return looking grim. Mike and Greg

say they can't tell how he died. Even if that isn't true, I'm glad they tell me no more. I'd rather not know. In usual circumstances I would collapse in a heap, but I can't. I have to be strong for this baby. Somehow that is exactly what I do.

Our beautiful friends over the river are a great support. I've been saying 'any day now' for almost five weeks. Being two weeks over due I'm a little impatient. I'm sure this baby must have waited until all the recent stress was over and for that I'm very grateful. All my check-ups are saying everything is fine, so I'm happy to keep waiting. The days go by and finally one evening, two and a half weeks overdue, I begin to feel slight contractions. All through the night I have mild to medium contractions. I wake on the morning of my twenty-ninth birthday in labour. With Ann unavailable I'm very relieved to call in Barbara, my back up midwife. Not only does she attend home births, Barbara is a hospital midwife with an enormous amount of experience which gives me confidence despite being an hour away from the closest hospital.

All day my contractions build. Mike and Barbara explain to Jemma what's happening. Barbara gives her a moist washer and shows Jemma to wipe my face. By 5 pm I'm exhausted and my contractions are intense. I think if I were at the hospital I would probably ask for pain relief despite my strong preference against the use of drugs during childbirth.

"I don't know if I can keep going," I tell Barbara.

"Everything is normal. You're doing very well."

"I wish I would go into second stage. I remember that was a lot easier."

Barbara has been massaging my tummy and putting me in a few different positions for a while. "We just need to try and turn the bub a little. He might be a touch posterior."

"Really?"

"That's ok. It's quite common. They often turn."

I don't know why, but I think to myself, If I'm not going into second stage, I will just push anyway. Doing so must be just enough to activate things. Suddenly, I have a huge contraction with an enormous urge to push. I can't help but push with every ounce of strength in my body.

"Oh, here's the head already!" Barbara exclaims.

"What's the baby doing?" Jemma asks.

"Coming out," Mike replies.

With the contraction stopping I have to wait for the next one. "Is he alright?" I ask.

"Yeah, he's fine," Mike says.

A few minutes later, with one more contraction, Lily is born. I hold her with joy and relief.
"Another girl," Mike says stroking her head, "This is your little sister Jemma. A little, baby girl."
Jemma sits in Mike's lap, in awe.
"Oh, what a relief. I can't believe how quick that was."
Barbara watches over us, making sure baby and I are both fine.
The months pass and Lily is growing well. Mike is working away at his brother's house but I'm determined to stay at home and not let Albert intimidate me. I put Lily in the pouch around my waist while Jemma and I feed the chooks and horses. Sitting in the paddock as the sun sets, the mist rises in the valley framed by the mountains beyond. We wander back to the cabin along the stony gravel driveway. I stoke up the fire and cook dinner. As usual I lie with the girls one under each arm reading a book as we all fall asleep.
I'm woken in the middle of the night with a loud bang. Immediately I know it's a gunshot. Quickly I go to the door making sure it's properly locked. I double check all the latches on the windows and ensure there are no gaps in the curtains. Returning to bed I watch over the girls as they sleep. I'm shaking but determined not to let that horrible man ruin our lives. I look at my girls. "What would I do if he came in?" I wonder helplessly. My thoughts go crazy. I try to make myself be strong. Eventually I breakdown. Tearfully I admit to myself how scared I am. I can't do this anymore. I feel an enormous sense of surrender towards myself, towards my own feelings of needing to be strong. I don't want to have to be strong anymore. With no more gunshots I eventually fall back to sleep. In the morning I pack our things and immediately take the girls to join Mike.
Spring arrives luring vibrant carpets of daffodils from their winter hibernation. Everywhere I look there's a sprinkling of yellow signalling a celebration of warmer weather. We have barbeques by the river, inviting neighbours, friends and family. As much as I try to enjoy it I'm becoming tired, mentally, emotionally and physically. Tired of living near a psychopath. Tired of having to start the generator for power. Tired of the extra work of my water saving twin tub washing machine. Tired of firing up the stove for hot water. Tired, tired, tired. But most of all, I am tired of trying to keep warm.
With dusk upon us I feed the chooks and the horses, and put their rugs on. Down the hill I see the lights of Mike's car approaching. Dinner is now eaten beneath a light powered by the generator without even a thought

of a candlelit dinner. An hour or two after dark I jump, once again, to the sound of gun shots vibrating through our cabin. Mike is fed up. So am I. Soon the phone rings. It's John from over the river. He too, has had enough of these gun shots sounding through the valley. It would be different if it were a responsible hunter but we all know this is intentional intimidation. "I'm coming over," he says.

I'm scared for John. Albert could be anywhere near the road letting off wayward shots. My heart is pounding hard. I sigh with relief when John's car pulls up at our cabin and he comes inside. Mike and John discuss the situation.

"I've told the police again but there's nothing they can do," complains Mike.

"Come on, let's go and try to see where he is," John says to Mike.

Despite my protest that it's not safe, they step out into the darkness. I hear more shots. "Oh, please don't let it be them." I pray. I'm a nervous wreck. I cannot handle this. On their return I curse them and tell them never to do that again!

During the next week I suggest we move back up North. Mike doesn't seem keen. All together we have been here for three and a half years now. Plenty of time to settle in and make strong connections with friends and family. But I feel like something has to give, that something is going to happen. I hate how I often feel tense, anxious and fatigued, and asthma is causing me more trouble than it has in a long time.

"Well just give me time to get this job finished," Mike relents after some strong convincing.

"Thank you," I say, hugging him.

My excitement doesn't mask the sorrow I feel leaving. I hate saying goodbye. Looking back at the past three and a half years I wonder what I was trying to prove. Somewhere in my life I had learned you need to be tough to endure whatever comes at you. To fight what's wrong and unjust. But I see now it was that brute determination that eventually made me crack. I realise I didn't want or need to be so strong all the time. That allowing ourselves to break down, to not be strong is in fact a form of inner strength. One of the most powerful kinds. While at times we need willpower, allowing that strength, wisdom and knowing to arise from within is so much more powerful.

13 A Place of Deep Love and Connection

It's now been three years since my severe reaction to the tick bites. Three long years that I've been suffering these horrendous symptoms. Each time I feel improvement and relief I trick myself into thinking I'm so much better. Well I am so much better. I'm no longer bed bound and wondering if I'm going to drop dead any minute. But in reality, I'm not healthy. I'm just less close to death than I was before. The burning, tingling and cramping in my muscles never lets up day or night especially down my right side. My symptoms still become much worse after eating and my whole chest fills with a burning sensation. I dread eating because of the pain but force myself to eat regular meals. I eat only three large meals a day without snacking to avoid the burning as much as possible. The heart palpitations and adrenalin are still constantly high but not as bad as they used to be.
I often wake during the night dripping in sweat, my pyjamas and sheets saturated. Every morning I wake up filled with dread and an agonising cramping discomfort in my belly where this lump still seems to be. I'm so forgetful and have serious brain fog, often just looking at something and soon wondering what I was about to do. Feeling jittery all the time, my nervous system still feels shot. I keep reminding myself that I'm so much better than I was, but I know there's still something seriously wrong. There *has* to be something, but I don't know what. I spend time each day working towards improving my overall health yet I'm so fed up with it. I just don't want to think about it anymore. I do my best to be open to whatever may help, but at the same time trying my hardest to ignore this agony and fill my life with as much peace and happiness as I can each day. Jemma's good friend is a member of the local longboard surfing club and she's very keen to join. Everyone is very welcoming and one member lends us a board to take home which the girls enjoy much more than short boards. Despite my aversion to competitions some of the members talk us into attending one of the weekend competitions down the coast. As we soon discover, rather than a competitive weekend, this is actually an excuse for surfers from all over the country to come together enjoying the surf shared meals, campfires, dancing and lots of good times. Oh, and of course the surfing as well. We enjoy a great weekend. I treasure every moment with my girls and everyone here, sharing in these simple pleasures and joys of life.

Di Ellis

I recently joined an A Capella singing group. I still can't believe that I seem to be able to sing a little. My whole life I've never been able to. It's only been spending time with Christian and Rose, singing along with their mantra meditations, that I've learnt how to hold a note. I'm no good at singing on my own but in a group with harmonies, it's magical. Cath, the leader of the choir has invited me to join her and another lady, Jenny, to sing as a trio at an Australia day event. I figure it's just a BBQ in the park and pretty casual so I should be right. That is until I discover it's a gala dinner with the Mayor. I am petrified. Well actually, I'm not. But I should be. I'm actually quite relaxed. But I shouldn't be. If I stop thinking, somewhere deep down, I am feeling relaxed and quietly confident. I don't know how or why, but I am. I guess learning to detach my emotions from unnecessary thoughts has been very beneficial in many unexpected ways. During the performance I'm on autopilot. I have no idea what I'm doing. Acting as though I'm a seasoned professional I don't think anyone would realise I'm so nervous. Everyone is thrilled with our performance. I'm laughing so much on the inside. Little does anyone know what a fluke that was. Just like the Kirtan chanting when I sing and drum with people, whether we perform on not, I feel a deep soul connection with those around me. We might have nothing in common in our day-to-day lives and may barely know each other, but we are taken beyond that to a place of deep love and connection. It's these connections which are keeping me going in life. Helping me to get through the underlying agony that persists in my body. Even if only for brief moments I'm able to free myself and feel pure joy, relief and happiness.

Ever since the liver cleanses, then the removal of my tooth, I've been glad to have so much energy. Relieved that I no longer feel so fatigued all the time as I did for so many years. Yet in its place this awful inability to sit still or truly relax drives me crazy. It's extremely frustrating. When the agitation stirs in my body it feels like being in a car that's in neutral with the accelerator down. In fact, that is how I feel all day every day. My mind is relaxed in neutral, but I just cannot relax my body no matter how hard I try or don't try. Over and over I question what the hell is going on. I know I've had massive trauma in my life but I also know what I'm experiencing is not simply in my mind. This is definitely a serious physical condition. But I don't know what to do about it and I hate that. There's a missing piece to this and I'm going to find it. I'm determined to regain my health one hundred percent.

I decide to order Dr Clark's VariGamma and an ozonator. I begin ozonating all of the water I drink. I also ozonate olive oil which Dr Clark says holds and distributes the ozone well in the body. Ozone being three oxygen molecules is very effective at killing bacteria by oxidizing it and blasting a hole in its cell wall. Shortly after taking the ozone I have very strong indigestion, like the burning sensations I still get after eating but much worse. The next morning when I wake up my right-hand side is tingling with pins and needles. I move around to get the circulation going. My right eye is lazy and puffy. I'm guessing the Lyme bacteria, which seem to have particularly affected my right side are dying due to the ozone.

The VariGamma is a computerized version of the zapper, which can be set specifically for every parasite, bacterium or virus. I also bought the computerized chips programmed with frequencies against Lyme disease and, for preventative measures, I also purchase the cancer chip. First trying the Lyme frequency card I have myself wired up. Anything to get rid of these Lyme symptoms. I feel the slight electric current coming through the wristbands. Very soon my chest is burning with feelings of indigestion and the tingling in my right foot is intense. Great! I know it's doing what it's meant to be doing. I've heard of warnings for people when they start any treatment for Lyme disease because of the herxheimer reaction which usually occurs when the Lyme bacteria are being killed off. Basically our body becomes burdened with the resulting die off. That seems to be exactly what's happening now as all my symptoms are heightened. This is great! Something is happening! Many people report a worsening in their symptoms which can show up in a huge variety of ways including headaches, joint, muscle and body pain, tingling, cramps, sore throat, fever, chills, sweating, nausea, brain fog, depression, anxiety and more.

Once again I notice some improvements, but unfortunately my excitement turns to disappointment as many of my symptoms persist. I plummet into confusion and despair over this nasty insidious disease. I wonder how I can ever possibly free myself of it. I see a television show with footage of a lady who was desperately unwell for a long time and eventually passed away. I listen to her broken-hearted mother telling her story of trying so desperately to help her daughter regain health. This beautiful mother is beside herself with grief and frustration due to the battle with medical authorities who ignored her daughter's plight. Oh how I know that frustration so well. Discussions about the tedious and fruitless struggle to regain health and the despair over the lack of recognition and medical assistance for Lyme disease in Australia raise awareness of the seriousness of this issue. Tears pour down my face. I wonder if some of the treatments I have used might have helped her daughter. Seeing footage of this sick woman in agony, lying in bed barely able to get up, I remember exactly what that felt like. It reminds me just how much I have improved despite the pain I'm still in and encourages me to keep going. For everyone else who is suffering I have to speak up. I make a commitment to sharing as much as I can the simple techniques which have helped me so much this far.

14 Shark Attack

It's nearing 6 am as the day begins to break. If predictions are correct it will be good surf this morning. I consider going out straight away but usually don't last too long if I haven't had breakfast. No, I'll cook up a quick feed first I think to myself. I hear a car going past. A neighbour, Steve, is off for his usual dawn surf. It's a bit creepy being in the water too early so I'm happy to give the sun a little time to rise above the horizon.

The ocean is smooth and glassy with lines of nicely-sized swell. I feel the call of the waves. Rough stones massage my feet as I walk down the dirt track towards Angourie Point. The path is criss-crossed with spider webs. I'm nearly at the bottom of the track when a local boy comes running up, "Don't go out there! There's a shark. There's a shark attack!"

"What's happened? Who is it?" asks another surfer nearby.

"Steve."

"Is there anyone with him?"

"Yeah, and Dad too," he says in between breaths.

"Is he alright?" I ask.

"Yeah, he's sitting on the beach," he points towards Back Beach. "I've gotta go tell the others not to go out."

With my first aid training flashing through my mind I run along the track through the bush towards Back Beach. My heart pounds as all sorts of terrible images come to mind. I pray that he's not too bad. Just as I reach the car park, Steve and his companions walk up the pathway.

I look him all over, "Are you ok?"

"Yeah, I'm ok." He turns his board towards me.

"Wholly crap!"

There's a huge semi-circular piece missing with jagged teeth marks along the edge. Fellow surfers and friends begin to gather around as Steve lifts the bottom of his knee high wet suit, revealing four or five small slashes on his thigh, each one about a centimetre long. We are all stunned.

"Geez, you can't even see any holes in your wetsuit," one surfer says, "It's like a razor blade has slashed through it."

A few drops of watery blood run down his leg. Despite the situation Steve seems fairly relaxed and jovial.

"How in the hell did it take such a big bite out of your board and only just scrape you like that?" asks a surfer.

"I was paddling for a wave and just as I went to get up it hit me from underneath. I went flying through the air."
"Must've scared the shit out of you?"
"Yeah, just a bit."
We all stand around Steve, dumbfounded, looking at him and his board in amazement.
"Well no bloody wonder he didn't want you. Stupid shark picked the skinniest bloke to take a bite from."
The jokes are flying thick and fast now. Not in a reckless, careless way, quite the opposite. The mateship is warming and I'm sure it has a calming effect on Steve.
"You'd better be careful. You're probably in a bit of shock," I warn.
"I think you've got a good reason to have the day off work today mate," one of the guys says as everyone begins to disperse.
"Don't tell Julia what happened. She won't let you go surfing again."
"You'll get whatever you want today, big fella. You'll be waited on hand and foot," trailed another voice.
Many people have gathered at the lookout. A surfer paddles out to Angourie Point to warn everyone there has been a shark attack on the other side of the headland. Most surfers come in but some remain.
"Look at those crazy bastards staying out there," someone says.
I watch them, admiring what a beautiful day it is. They're catching some awesome waves. My mind is ticking over. I've never heard of two attacks in one day. Or at the same place. I can't possibly be considering going for a surf? Can I? I don't feel fearful at all about the idea. Really, we are all taking the risk every day when we go surfing. Maybe there is *less* chance of being bitten now.
"I don't know. I don't think the shark would have liked that mouthful of foam," I say to one of the women observing. "I doubt he would be quick to do it again."
"You'd still be crazy to be out there," she replies. "Your children are pretty old now aren't they? I guess they don't really need you anymore."
I look at her in confusion. It takes me a moment to realise she is being sarcastic. Little does she know how much the fear of losing people has affected my life, or that the desire to be here for my children is what drives me to hold on to my own life every day.
I question myself over and over, "How on earth am I not fearful of a shark? Why am I feeling this way? Have I become reckless?" No. I don't feel reckless. I just don't feel scared. And I don't want fear to stop me from living my life any more. Also, when I'm in the water my body feels

so good. I'd rather go for a surf than go back and sit at home. I don't mention it to anyone, but I know I will go for a surf soon. I wouldn't go out at Back Beach where the attack was, but Angourie Point feels okay. I have so much faith in my instincts now. Every time I have ignored them in the past I have made a mistake or something bad has happened. But now I listen, trusting them fully and know everything will be fine.

I wait a little while for most people to leave. I really don't want anyone thinking I'm reckless. I don't think they would quite understand if I say, 'Oh it's okay, if I was going to die it would have been during the last year or two when I was really sick. I know that when your time is up it's up, and I know it's not my time yet'. How can I tell them I've been on an amazing inner journey and have learnt to trust my instincts so much that I live my life by them now. They are telling me everything will be fine. I know this with every cell of my body.

As I enter the water many thoughts are going through my mind. There are only three or four locals out, it's a beautiful day and the waves are fantastic. Not too big, but big enough to have a lot of fun and one of my best surfs at the Point. We all discuss why we believe it's safe enough to be out here. I'm quite surprised to feel completely at ease during my whole time in the water. That is, apart from the surprise a turtle gives me when he surfaces next to me. How lucky am I to be out here? I cherish every moment. A couple of hours of being in the water and I begin to feel the jittery weakness through my spin and back, my body telling me it's had enough. I catch a wave, feeling very content.

While I'm still on my healing journey I have discovered we all have an incredible gift of knowing; that voice or feeling within that says something just is or maybe isn't right. That innate sense of intuition we are all born with is one of the most powerful tools we will ever have, at our disposal every moment of every day of our lives. What may be good for one may not be good at all for another. But when we learn to listen to that voice within, it will guide and assist us to navigate through any challenges and steer us toward a path of joy and happiness … if we will only learn to listen, but most importantly, trust in this process.

15 Allowed to Love

The surf feels like my safe haven. The only place where I truly feel relaxed in my body. Often people are friendly but happy to keep to themselves. This provides an environment with no need to talk, no need to meet any expectations. Just being. Sitting, watching, and waiting for a wave to roll in. There is also a sense of security with people nearby. I realise how important it is during a healing journey to have a place you can go to feel relaxed, peaceful and accepted.

The cool gentle and constant movement rocks and eases my body. I know people see me looking fit, surfing and having so much fun regularly, but they have no idea the torment and pain I feel within and I have no intentions of letting them see it again. I keep up the façade of who I want to be. I know I will grow into this person someday. Somehow.

Often in the surf I see him, drawn into his world by those deep dark eyes. Each time I feel invited into his life though, he soon shuts down closing me out again. I then chastise myself for falling into old patterns. Well I guess they aren't *old* patterns. To my frustration it's an ongoing pattern. Or maybe I'm attracted to people who in some ways are just like me. When I was young, in nearly all of my relationships my feelings overwhelmed me and I ran away. By the time I realised what I'd done it was too late.

When I was seventeen my first boyfriend, bless his heart, was a radio announcer just like my birth father. My mother too was seventeen when she met my father. I knew nothing about either of them when I was that age, so how I recreated that pattern in my life I have no idea. No wonder I had so many strange feelings I couldn't understand or cope with. In confusion and despair I shut down my feelings and ran away. By the time I realised what a mistake that was it was too late. Unfortunately I didn't learn though and repeated this mistake a number of times. Now I don't really know what is happening between my friend and I. Maybe I'm attracted to people who won't let me get close to them, addicted to relationships that simply won't work. I don't know, but I do know I cannot run away this time. I need to try as hard as I can to stand steady and work through these feelings, dissolving these negative patterns once and for all.

While deep down I know I'm not ready for a relationship, I miss having a partner to love and share my life with. I notice that each time I set intentions about having a relationship or opening up to welcome love into my life I have a feeling like I'm being selfish and I tell myself, 'No, I need to keep my health a priority.' Lying down practising some breathing exercises I tune into my body and how I'm feeling. I begin to realise that I've had a long-held belief that I have to choose one or the other. My health or love. Every time I concentrate on overcoming this belief thoughts enter my mind about the separation from my mother when I was born. I can see myself. I'm looking down from a corner of the ceiling. I can see the hospital room and the doctor wearing gloves and a mask. And being taken straight from my mother without her ever seeing me. This image I've had many times in the past.

The pieces are beginning to come together. Right from when I was born I learnt that if I wanted to survive I had to accept that I would not receive the love and nurturing that I so longed for. My first experiences of deep love were also some of my most horrific. Being snatched quickly away from my mother before I could even take my first breath. The umbilical cord cut, my only connections to life and love up to this point severed in the same moment. The reason why I panicked and ran away from my early relationships finally dawns on me. The deepest cellular memory of love I hold within is directly related to my deepest fear and trauma. The trauma of my birth. Struggling to take my first breath while being torn from my mother. Each time I felt love on a deep level the cellular memory in my body was triggered and an immediate fear and panic for my life set in, so I ran away. I'm finally gaining understanding of the confusion within.

I'm no longer astounded by all of these feelings and memories that come to me from when I was so young or even in the womb. It's just another part of my life now. I realise we all have unresolved feelings, whether or not there has been a big or traumatic separation. Some of these feelings may be created during what many may call a routine birth. For others, seemingly insignificant events may have had great impact on them as a very small child. It's just my unique set of circumstances that has driven me to explore so rigorously where these feelings are coming from. But no matter where such feelings originate, allowing them and feeling them while moving forward in our lives is vitally important.

I remind myself it's our birth given right to experience deep unconditional love and nurturing, as well as having a strong and healthy body. Even just saying that to myself I experience an enormous amount of relief. I feel my whole body relaxing and releasing on a deep level. I've always been able to feel deep love and I've always known that I deserve to have love in my life, but actually feeling and believing that on a cellular level is a different thing.

I'm realising how deeply the memories held within our body affect us. I can so easily go back to the womb. Back to a heavenly place where I'm bathed in the deepest most incredible love whether from my mother or a connection to a higher source. But I'm finding that depth of love so difficult to sustain in my daily life and I don't know why. My ill-health and the events around it have been very traumatic particularly for Jemma. She still has difficulty coping. I'm certainly having difficulty coping with her, especially while deep down I'm still very unwell. This leads to one of the darkest moments of my life, when I reach out for help from her father. I ask him to come and take her to help sort things out. I'm later told I brought this whole situation on myself.

I also reach out to a counsellor to provide help for us all in this situation. To my horror after all I have given, heart and soul to this beautiful being, I am belittled and told to go home and have a hot bath and a cup of tea. This man, this supposed counsellor who is paid to support people who come to him may as well have just stabbed me in the heart. I walk out of that office with an understanding of the helplessness and depths people reach when they commit suicide. I really don't know why I have such a strong connection to life, for after all that I have been through you would think I would consider harming myself. But I don't.

Jemma, against my wishes is no longer in my care. It seems she is welcomed into a new life and told to forget about her old one. I know I have done so well to get her this far and she is now a beautiful young woman of nearly seventeen, but for things to happen this way is totally devastating. One of the reasons I held onto life so dearly has now been taken from me. With every cell I know I have given everything I can possibly give without surrendering my own integrity. I have worked through so many mixed up feelings in myself over the years. I have always tried to sort out problems. I tried to be there for everybody. I tried to give everything I could. I tried to be this. I tried to be that. The deep loss that I feel is intense. The daughter I had is no longer there, not even to speak to. I know I did everything I could do. I could not fix anything else. I could not change anything and now I cannot do anything to take these feelings away. I've finally reached the bottom of the barrel. Deeply seated within me, beneath the loss, I find a fear so intense, so primal, nothing can hide it. Nothing can make it feel better.

Everything in my life that usually brings me joy suddenly seems completely empty and lifeless. Where did all the happiness go? Each day

I don't know what to do to make myself feel any joy. This illness feels like it has consumed me. This is the deepest darkest grief I have ever felt and it's relentless. I know the only thing I can do is surrender completely to this feeling. I go about each day feeling like a zombie. I observe my thoughts. Observe how my body is feeling. How I am feeling no matter how much I hate it. Finally I realise the only way I can deal with these awful feelings in me every day is to pretend they are my friend. Instead of falling into dread every time these feelings arise I pretend they are there for me, like a lifelong companion always by my side. Within a very short time I suddenly notice they are completely gone. 'Where did they go?' I wonder. 'How did they go?' I don't know. But they just aren't there anymore. My whole body feels lighter. My whole life, once again feels lighter. Somehow as a society we have learnt or been conditioned to shut down our feelings. In doing so, we often don't know how to feel anymore or what to do with those feelings. There is a gift in learning to feel our feelings.

With more important realisations I notice how much I've given in my life. Given to be wanted. To be needed. To be accepted. Given people what they want, but never really known what I want. I could keep doing that all my life, yet still it may never be enough. I hit the point where I realise that if you are at peace within yourself, by yourself, there is nothing to fix. Nothing to do. Nothing to make 'right'. Just loving is enough. Just being is enough. I knew I could not talk anymore. I could not listen anymore. I could not give anymore. I was empty. I could do nothing but be. Be there, be love, be me.

Now I notice if I'm not standing strong in my own energy, if I'm out of balance or jeopardising myself for others, I can see how it has an immediate effect on the energy of people around me and the way they relate to me. For a long time I've also observed the effect on my own energy when I'm around other people. Occasionally I've noticed how depleted or anxious I may feel around someone, even if on the surface all seems to be good. At other times there may be people who are not very friendly but for some reason I feel comfortable around them. Extraordinary exchanges of energy can occur within a seemingly simple interaction. I'm learning to centre my energy at all times. If I forget and allow my energy to be affected by other people or to go astray, I bring my focus back to myself, to my breath and to my body. Usually this allows me to feel good within myself no matter what someone else might be saying, thinking, feeling or even projecting towards me.

Louise Hay talks of parasites representing giving our power away to others. Letting them take over. I see how much I have done this in my life even at times when I thought I was being strong. When we've had traumas, illness or simply just criticism and lowered self-esteem we often become much more vulnerable to this. We doubt ourselves. We think other people have more authority or their views hold more substance. When feeling this way, we may as well plug a power cord from ourselves into that other person or people.

So many times I've reached amazing places of peace and harmony within myself only to later wonder how much more of life's 'crap' is there? How much more am I supposed to work through? Why can't I just get on with living life? Yet each time I worked through any difficulties I found myself closer to my authentic self, experiencing deeper feelings of joy, peace and happiness within. Bringing deeper meaning to my life. I'm not sure how, but somehow I know these processes are connecting that deep love I feel when I revisit my time in the womb, to my daily existence now.

When Jemma was little she questioned everything, asking me, "Why, why, why?"

"What you doin' Di?" she would ask in her beautiful little three-year-old voice, head tilted looking at me curiously.

"Hanging out the washing."

"Why?"

"So the clothes will dry."

"Why."

"So you can have warm clothes to wear."

"Why?"

"Because I love you and I want you to be comfortable."

In the end the answer always came back to love. At the core of all of our feelings there is either love, fear or both. Beneath all positive feeling is love. Love for ourselves. Love for others or love for our home, land or environment. Beneath all negative feeling is fear. Beneath all anger, hatred or grief is the fear for ourselves, fear for others or fear for our home, land or environment. Asking Jemma's 'why' question about anything in our lives is an easy way to come to this conclusion. Many of the processes in our body causing us to feel fear and negative feelings are the same processes through which we feel love and all associated positive feelings.

If we block out our feelings of fear, grief, hatred and anger we are also blocking the pathways in our body which help us to feel happiness, gratitude, joy, love and peace. In turn this may cause the development of many different illnesses. It always comes back to allowing our inner feelings while making a conscientious effort towards positive thoughts, intentions and affirmations. In doing this I'm still so surprised how easily feelings of grief, anger and hurt can transform into feelings of love, joy and peace. When those negative feelings arise, no matter where you are or what you are doing, just acknowledge them and allow them while you go about your business. If you're in a private place and feel comfortable to do so allow those feelings to their full depths. Try not to expect an immediate positive transformation as these processes often happen spontaneously in their own time. Be open to all possibilities and trust the blocked energy in your body is moving and releasing simply by giving acknowledgment to these feelings within yourself.

Looking back over my life I can see that many people and circumstances have reflected what was actually happening within me, mirroring parts of myself. I had been taught this and read about it, but I wondered how it could possibly be. How could someone so cruel and malicious as Albert represent a part of me? I am certainly nothing like him, or so I thought. I can see it clearly now though. There were parts of myself that I was rejecting. I did not want the sides of myself that were hurting so deeply. I would have been happy if that part of me died, if it just went away and disappeared. But that part of me also held a huge amount of love, a large part of my heart and soul. It seemed as though Albert was wanting to get rid of me, just as I was wanting to get rid of those parts of myself. And it was he who triggered the need for me to go deep within myself, to heal past wounds that had been affecting my life without me realising it. Had that not have happened I may not have found those incredible depths of love within myself.

Though it is very difficult not to have resentment towards my girls' father, I know that without even realising it, he stopped me from compulsively giving, leaving myself constantly empty and not receiving. I would have given myself for my girls. Often I have had feelings that my adopted mother died because she gave too much of herself. Gave too much of herself to me. Had she not given so much of her life-force, her energy to me, she may not have died. Through my own ill-health I now know that statement to be false, but with a touch of truth. It is not that she gave herself to me or anyone else, it is that while she was giving to others somewhere along the way she lost herself, her spirit, her soul. I'm not sure how, but somehow in her passing I feel she was going back home to herself, to wherever her spirit had gone. On the other hand, my birth mother who lost everything had nothing left to hold on to except herself.

In doing so she has shown me how to survive, how to hold on to my own life-force and to be strong in myself, no matter what happens.

I know I have been very strict with my girls, some may even say I have deprived them as their father at times thought. But instead of letting them be taken away with the superficial meaningless things in life, I've always reminded them what's important. So many times I didn't let them have television, computer games or lollies at the shops. They just had to find something for themselves to do or just do nothing. I wanted them to be happy and content within themselves. In the same way that I did my best to teach them, I'm teaching myself. I'm so proud of the strength I have found within myself. I've learnt to be very stoic and able to detach when need be, but in a way that takes me closer to soul and spirit without closing off my heart.

It's been a challenge to accept that life is not 'happening' to me, but rather is responding to me and what is held within. But I now know it to be true. This is what this healing journey has taught me. It takes willpower to change negative thoughts and patterns, and to let go of what you think you want. To be open and responsive to what you really need for deep fulfilment. I play and experiment with my own emotions at times, watching how they change by changing my thoughts, then observing where these changes will lead me and what they will manifest in my life. If I don't like what I'm feeling I change my thoughts until I find a thought pattern that is leading me to a positive place. This I have learnt is actually changing the neural pathways in our brain. At times, for curiosity or if need be, I will venture into a place of darkness within myself to see where it might go, but I don't usually stay there for too long unless there is something positive to be gained; either a release of blocked energy in the body or an awareness around an issue.

If you have a traumatic thought or feeling, sit with it briefly. Where do you feel this in your body? Focus your awareness and attention to this area with nice full relaxed breaths and allow the energy to shift. You may feel a release or softening. If you feel at ease to do so you may like to explore more emotions or thoughts around this issue, always bringing your awareness to your body and breath to allow any shifts of energy to occur. However, if your instincts are setting off an alarm bell listen to this. You may be rehashing an emotional hurt which may be better left in the past. There are times when a movie or a conversation can trigger our thoughts to lead us into a negative and upsetting thought pattern, possibly a neural pathway which is better left to fade away. This is when we may need to walk out of the movie or change the conversation. If you feel them having a negative affect on you be assertive to stop those negative thoughts and create positive thoughts and conversations which make us feel better within ourselves. In turn we are creating new neural pathways which will automatically create more positive thoughts.

For six months or so I've barely heard from Jemma. Now at seventeen and getting ready for her debutante ball, I'm delighted she has asked me to come. Her hair tied back into flowing curls, she's absolutely beautiful. A stunning turquoise dress compliments her curvaceous figure. She is glowing, loving every moment as she spins and twirls around the dance floor. When it comes time for the special person's dance Jemma makes her way over to our table where she is expecting Harley, her good friend, to accompany her. She doesn't know I've secretly been taking lessons to learn all the moves. She signals for him to join her but he doesn't move. Instead he looks at me and grins as I stand up.

In protest, yet smiling, Jemma says, "But you don't know it."

"Oh well," I reply.

We make our way to the dance floor and I take her hands asserting my male position, as the instructor's words run through my mind. The music starts and I lead her strongly into every step. I see her trying to hold back her smile. Forward and back we go, around and around. Whilst others, still having a great time but have not learnt the part, fumble and laugh their way through, Jemma and I float effortlessly around the dance floor.

"How am I going?" I ask with a grin.

"You've had lessons!" she says with a big smile on her face.

The happiness within me is immense.

Di Ellis

16 The Beauty Beneath Life and Death

"Did you see that one Mum?" calls Jemma, paddling back out after catching a good wave. Surfing with my girls is like being in heaven. Jemma's surfing has taken off. She catches wave after wave, often putting her arms up to the sky in delight. I return the gesture with pride. Lily decides she wants me to double with her on the longboard, something we've never done before. Floating about we wait for the right wave. Arms and legs flapping, we feel the board picked up by the momentum of the wave. As we attempt to stand up I'm hit in the face with Lily's backside. Somehow we manage to get to our feet. We are up for a few seconds until Lily overbalances, slaps me in the face and we fall into the water laughing so hard we can barely breathe. I instruct Lily to wait to let me get up first and gain control of the board. Finally we master it and glide many times wobbling and giggling along the waves. Jemma catches a wave by our side, the three of us riding all the way from out the back in to the shore. This is joy!
Seeing dolphins further down the beach I paddle in their direction. Blissfully I watch them swimming in the waves towards me, under and around, jumping out of the water as they please. Excitement rushing through my body, I stand on my board and dive into the water. "I'm out very deep," I think to myself. "On my own at Back Beach where the shark attack was." Pushing those thoughts out of my mind I surface, take a breath and swim underwater with the dolphins. Fins are rising and submerging all around me. Their grey skin gleams and shines as they come up for a breath, the sound of air rushing through their blowholes. One comes straight for me before going under, then surfaces again directly in front of me barely a metre away. This moment stands still. Her deep dark eye looks into mine, deep into my soul. These majestic creatures surround me as I giggle like a little girl. I float for a moment paddling on my back before rolling and tumbling under the water, the soft warmth caressing my body.
This deep love I feel for nature and all within has been warming to my spirit. I have no doubt it has nurtured, nourished and healed my soul. The ocean and national park nearby are filled with an abundance of wildlife. I find myself drawn into their world, happy to escape my own. I'm fascinated by the bizarre and intimate encounters I have with many creatures. Beautiful ancient looking lizards, the bearded dragons and water dragons sunning themselves on the dunes while overlooking the

ocean. Many snakes including the harmless carpet pythons, the intriguing and a touch terrifying venomous red belly black, and brown snakes. The dolphins and their babies. Gannets, the enormous sea birds gliding and skimming across the water just metres away. Snorkelling on days with no surf when a stunningly majestic garden of vibrant coloured sea plants and creatures reveals itself hidden beneath Life and Death, the rock shelf which so effortlessly traps surfers when the waves are big. I look around and absorb all of earth's incredible beauty and energy, filling and arousing all of my senses.

No matter what it is in life that provides this relief, these moments of joy, they are so incredibly important and never, ever to be underestimated. Any time you are feeling upset, let down by others or confused with the world, find your own way of connecting with nature. Whether it's watching a sunrise or sunset, the stars and the moon, or sitting in a park or tree. Feel that oneness with the earth, with the universe and allow it to diminish the conflicts and problems you may be experiencing. Allow those problems to dissolve into menial illusions even if only temporarily until you find a way to resolve them with ease ... or maybe, just maybe the universe might do it for you!

Now after being so incredibly unwell I feel so much gratitude for every small or large thing; a flower growing unexpectedly in the bush, a catch up with a friend and even just paddling out in the water on my board whether or not I catch a wave. It has taken this horrid illness for me to truly understand, to the depths of my soul, the practice of gratitude in the now, in this present moment. By being grateful for all of the simple things, we have at our disposal an infinite and eternal stream of joy.

I know the excitement and gratitude I feel when catching a wave or doing something physical is not only because it's fun, but also because I'm just so grateful to have regained so much health. But I wonder how long it will last. There is a weariness or maybe a knowingness that my body just can't keep going like this. Despite all of the learnings and enjoyment I am experiencing the constant deep agony screaming from within is haunting and never ending.

Lately I've been noticing a small scaly itching spot on my back and I figure I'd better do something about it. I use an ointment called Black Salve which destroys cancerous cells while leaving healthy cells alone. I've used the salve successfully on moles with some of them being eaten away while others are untouched. I do a few applications over a few days. To my horror the affected area is much bigger than I realized. In panic I wipe the ointment over a very large area. If this is cancer I want to get rid of it.

Now! I hold off using pain killers. I want to be able to feel what is happening in my body. Strangely the last two times I've put on the salve, within minutes I've experienced a burning, tingling, itchy sensation going right through me to the area of my liver, under my ribs on the right-hand side where I've had so much cramping over the years. I wonder if the cancer has spread internally and the salve is eating its way through.

I try to sleep during the night, but I'm in far too much pain. Fearful of what's happening I wash off the salve. Again, I resist taking pain killers so I can feel what's going on in my body. The pain going through to the area of my liver continues on and off as the action of the salve persists. The next day I make an appointment with a doctor who practises complementary medicine and I hope he's open to what I've done. I make it very clear that I'm not going through conventional methods of testing and treatment and I'm so relieved and grateful when he is supportive. He says that he can't agree with what I've done, but he can monitor my situation. His caring helpful manner calms me. He thinks the pain in the liver area is only referred nerve pain from my back but still suggests I have an ultrasound. To my frustration it doesn't give me any answers.

For days the pain is intense. A ten centimeter circular area of my back has been eaten away. I feel as though I've been shot in the back. I wonder what in the hell is happening with me and what in the hell I've done to myself. Surely I can't have friggin' cancer as well as Lyme? I knew I've had a lot of underlying problems even before the Lyme, but I don't need this. I think about my grandfather. One person who I haven't forgiven. The one person who I know I hold very deep hatred and resentment for. The man who abandoned my mother when she was pregnant with me. The deacon of the church who forbade my grandmother from keeping me when she so desperately wanted to.

I figured he died many years ago and I didn't know him, so there was no need for me to think about him or try to resolve anything concerning him. As thinking about him caused me pain, the less I thought about him the better. I know now that I've been very wrong about this. I know my deep-seated anger and resentment towards my grandfather is an underlying cause of this cancer. I also know that forgiving my grandfather is the most important thing that I need to do for myself. I need to release this pattern which I have obviously inherited. My grandfather died from cancer of the spine.

I feel angry when I think about forgiving him, really angry. I don't want to forgive him! I realize I *want* to hate him. I *really* want to hate him. How can I possibly forgive someone who I hate so much? But I need to. Not for him, but for myself. I don't want to do anything for him, but I have to do it for myself. I go within and wonder how I can possibly find feelings of forgiveness for him within myself. Immediately the answer is clear to me. I have an image in my mind. He is maybe four or five years old. He is being chastised once again. His spirit is crushed. His soul broken. Immediately I feel a deep love and compassion for him. I want to hold him and love him. I want to hold and love that part of him that is now me. That quarter of me that has developed from his genes, the part of me that I hated and wanted to die, which I suddenly realize is the part of me that *was* dying. I don't need to love the part of him that I felt was so evil. In fact I now see that I wanted to hate him because I never wanted to say that behavior is okay, because it wasn't and never will be. I realize I do unconditionally love who he was in his soul, and that little boy is now a part of me.

I'm amazed and shocked at what the salve has done. You can see all the contours and patterns where the cancer has been eaten away, some areas shallow, some deeper. There are even spots where it seems roots were growing. I realize I was quite foolish putting the salve on so liberally. I was in such a panic to get rid of any cancer but wonder if it was worth the damage I've done to my body. I seriously consider the possibility that the cancer has spread. I think back to over ten years ago when I first noticed tingling in my right hand and foot. The cancer may have already begun then. That was just after the trouble with my tooth began. The nerve trouble. The cancer. The dead tooth. All on my right side. Damn it, I knew of the connection with dead teeth and cancer twenty years ago. Naturally I'm worried. I'm careful and cautious, but I will not change my treatment plan. I have to keep moving forward.

Over the following weeks I do very little other than tend to my back helping it to heal. I begin making all sorts of anti-cancer concoctions and take pickings from our local communal garden, all beautifully fresh and nutritious organic food. Each bite I can feel the goodness filling my body. I know that if I hadn't been looking after myself and eating so well for many years I may not be walking or even alive. Come to think of it, if it weren't for the Lyme disease I certainly wouldn't have found and used all the simple and wonderful treatments that are effective against Lyme and cancer. How ironic it all is. When going for a walk, each step that I take across the boulders on the beach I feel the muscles along my spine working to keep me balanced. Each step I feel the solid rough strength of rock beneath my feet. I love every step I take.

It's been six weeks and the deep gouges taken out of my back are still healing but I'm determined to go in the Australian Longboard Titles, which are on in a few days. The first two rounds I do well and get into the semi-final, but unfortunately nerves get the better of me and I don't quite land the end of the best wave I catch. I'm a bit disappointed. When I'm free surfing I make waves like that all the time. But overall I come fifth in Australia for my age group so I'm very happy with that! Not that there are really all that many in my age group. Most of all I'm with a great bunch of people at a beautiful beach having a fantastic time. What more can I ask for?

Well there is one more thing I'm asking for. Back at the camping ground I'm tending to my back. There's one small deeper area which still hasn't healed. In fact it's growing larger and it's really worrying me. I'm shit scared actually. There's one voice telling me it's fine, I've just aggravated it surfing. The other fearful voice telling me it may be very fast growing cancer.

I think deep down I know it's fine, but once again I find myself saying, "I intend to be really healthy and get to the bottom of any health problems, bla bla bla bla blaaaa."

I'm sooo sick of saying this! Why is my body always screaming for attention? If it's not one thing it's something else. Overall my health seemed to be improving consistently, but enough already, I'm so sick of this shit! What is it that I'm not getting?

The fear that this cancer has created within me is deep. Therefore I know whatever it is that I need to work through is deep. I cannot run away from it. I cannot avoid it. I cannot turn to remedy after remedy. It's within me and I know I need to surrender to the fear, go down into it, feel it and listen to it.

"What is so deep within me, making me fearful of my own survival all the time?"

The answer comes to me straight away. I have an image of being in the womb. I hate my mother for not wanting me. I hate myself for being there and ruining her life. I can feel that I made a choice to close off the part of me that needed nurturing. I knew I would be able to nurture and give, but I chose not to be nurtured. That was too painful. I feel as though my mother closed off the part of her that craved to nurture and give, for that was too painful. Instead she chose to be nurtured. It seems we are completely opposite, but exactly the same.

I realize there are a few more people who I need to forgive. I'm so angry about this! I don't want to do this shit anymore. I just want to enjoy my life, be happy and forget all this stuff. I don't want to forgive them. How can I forgive people who show no remorse or compassion for hurtful actions they may have taken and *still* take, whether it be through ignorance or other? How can I forgive the deepest of wounds struck through my child? The sort of wound I could not escape from for she is part of both of us?

A friend recently returned one of Louise Hay's books which I haven't looked at for a long time. I close my eyes and open the book randomly pointing to a paragraph. I do this at times with any book if I want some guidance or direction. *Be willing to allow the changes to happen when they come up in your life. Be aware that where you DO NOT WANT TO CHANGE is exactly the area where you NEED to change the most.* I feel angry just reading this. Really, really angry! Visions of ripping this book to pieces come to my mind. But this is exactly what Louise is saying. I know I have to surrender. I have to do what I have to do. I don't want to. But I have to. How can I forgive? How? Especially when I know the same hurt keeps happening if I give it the chance? I have shut this out of my life to stop that hurt happening. I don't want to do this! But I think of the cancer and I know I have to.

I don't know what to do, but I shut my eyes and surrender. I make myself surrender and listen to my inner self. Before long I am back in the womb again. I fear for my life. I cannot stand everything that is going on; the fighting, the drama and the fear. I don't know exactly what is happening around me and my mother but I am very clear about the feelings of the events that are occurring. My mother is completely distraught, beside herself with fear and grief for her baby, her lover, and her family. Crushing feelings of abandonment, confusion and fear fill both of us. I can't handle it. I shut out the feelings in my body. I shut everything out, including my mother's love. So much so that dare I say it, I want to be given away. I want to be away from all of this. Well I got away from it, just as I'm away from it now, but it's still affecting me.

What else can I possibly do to release this pain? I have tried and tried and tried. Obviously what I'm doing is not working. So what if I *could* handle things, if I *was* strong enough, what would I have done? If I *could* forgive, what would I have done? I would have loved my mother anyway. Despite everything that was going on. Despite what she may or may not have done to try to get rid of me. No matter what our relationship is like now. I visualize her soul. I visualize loving her beneath all of the external circumstances. Immediately an enormous amount of tension releases from my body, just like a switch has been turned off. Being able to love, allowing myself to love regardless, is an enormous relief.

I realize a lot of inner tension has, to a degree, been created by feeling I needed to hold back my love. I don't feel the need to express that love now, but allowing myself to just feel it even if I wasn't supposed to, is a blissful relief in my body. I suddenly realize how all that tension has been a defense in my body, which has hurt me so much. I see how much guilt I have felt without even realizing it, just for being born, just for wanting to love. But no more. From now on it's just positive affirmations. I approve of myself. I love myself! Just as Louise Hay has always said. I see that the love of self is often hidden beneath negative feelings that we don't want to feel, such as grief, pain and fear. When these feelings arise remind yourself to be brave and gently explore into them with the intention of finding and embracing a deeper love for yourself. Doing so is an integral part of the healing process.

Loving myself is wonderful but I'm tired of doing this life thing alone. So if I learn to love myself unconditionally doesn't that mean my beautiful soul mate will magically appear? Or am I cursed to be a spinster for the rest of my life as the years disappear? I've done all the inner work, so why doesn't he just appear? There have at times been men come in and out of my life who I think I'm going to fall madly in love with, but I realize later it's just a story in my mind and nothing even comes of it. Since my marriage break up, one short summer romance evolved but went no further. I now find myself pining for someone, wondering if something could be. I want to turn my feelings off. All my old tricks come out. All the strategies to avoid the feelings I'm having. Distraction techniques, suppression and avoidance, and the biggest and best of them all; the complete shut down my heart trying-not–to-feel-anything-at-all trick. I want to run away, just like I did in my late teenage years galloping on my horse Cobba, letting him go and go. The wind in our hair, tears down my face, running away from the fear and hurt of relationships. But I'm too old and exhausted to keep running now. I *know* this must be happening for a reason. Time to go within and listen … *again*!

"I surrender! I will do whatever I have to do," I say opening my arms to the sky. I accept how I'm feeling. I allow the deep dark sinking feeling in my belly. I notice exactly where it is and how it feels in my body. I realize once again, that I have a deep feeling of grief that I will not be able to have the love in my life that I crave. I surrender to these feelings and breathe. I listen to my body and my inner self. My birth parents come to my mind. Am I ever going to be able to shake this curse? What now I wonder? All right I will listen! I bring my awareness within my body. I allow my inner self to show me what I need to know. I am back in the womb again. I know this story. I have been here so many times before.

These feelings of not being able to have the love that I crave fill me. They fill my mother. My mother is filled with grief because she cannot have the man she loves. Are these my feelings or her feelings I wonder? Have I been carrying my mother's grief all my life?

I sit with my feelings, allowing them to guide me. I become aware of how many times I've been in a situation where I care deeply for a man and feel I have to hide my feelings. That's exactly what my mother had to do. Surely my whole belief system and the way I function around relationships have not been formed from what I learnt in the womb? There's no other answer. All these thoughts and beliefs have been locked inside my whole life. No matter what I've learnt in over forty years from the world around, those underlying beliefs are what have been running the show. How can I change this? How can I free myself from these chains? A voice runs through my mind, "The truth will set you free," followed by Louise Hay's words. "Cancer is a deep secret or grief eating away at the self."

How will the truth set me free? What the heck are these thoughts coming into my mind? What are you on about now? I ask myself. I shut my eyes and feel. I observe the thoughts coming into my mind and the feelings in my body. What I used to work through in a breath session for one and a half hours with Anne now takes me about 2 minutes, but still after all these years I have a feeling as though I need to hide away. That I need to hide the truth as though my life depended on it.

Well I guess my life did depend on it when my mother was seventeen and she found out she was pregnant with me. In those days an unwed mother was unacceptable, shameful and hidden away, and often the baby was taken from them. Though it is something I have never seen expressed I can feel my mother's pain, her grief and despair. Why am I carrying this? It's like an energetic umbilical cord that has never been cut, draining the life-force from me. My mother told me she was never going to keep me, but I think back to my conversation with my aunt who told me differently. "You know, your mother was planning on keeping you. She was knitting clothes for you, you know. It was when your mother was around eight months pregnant they talked her into giving you up."

All these years later while the information my aunt had given me helped so much to make sense of the feelings I was having on a conscious level, I realise now, hidden within my subconscious, within my body, remain the energetic remnants of those hidden secrets. Those suppressed feelings of intense love, lust, shame, hurt and despair. It must have been an awful nightmare for my mother. Maybe for my father also. Imagine my grandfather's shame; an upstanding member of the community, deacon of the church. I can sense his fury. I doubt he knew the full truth. But what if the real truth was unconditional love. If the truth behind all of life is unconditional love? Is that not what my grandfather devoted his life towards – the love of God. All encompassing, all forgiving? What if even though my mother made a mistake, what if it was a good mistake and she was embraced and supported just the same. Imagine how she would have felt. How I would have felt. How would I feel now if there was acceptance rather than shame. Forgiveness rather than judgement. Love rather than anger and hatred. I would feel like I could breathe. Like I was allowed to be alive, allowed to thrive!

One day during the time of my breath sessions with Anne I was imagining the love that was present when I was conceived. Even if the act of my conception was not by the consent of my mother, I wanted to find the deepest level of love, even if only on the spiritual plane, which enabled the conception of a baby. To my surprise I had a vision of my mother and father walking hand in hand along a grassy field. Even more surprisingly in an unguarded moment, my vision was confirmed. At this moment I knew without doubt that I have been accessing knowledge from another dimension.

I'm at home listening to the Hay House World Summit. Hearing all of the speakers I feel a huge relief, as though I'm part of a community where I feel 'normal'. I relate so deeply to all of the information and wisdom being shared. I hear the voice of Tenzin Wangyal Rinpoche. "Every single pain you experience in your life, you do not want to waste them. No matter how strong it is, no matter how threatening it is, it is absolutely an opportunity for you to grow. Every spiritual master, their pain has been their awake call, their path, their means of transformation and opportunity."

In hearing this I have a profound moment of awakening. An instant transformation from being a victim of a relentless series of unfortunate events, to the master of an incredible inner journey. Suddenly I feel like a strong warrior woman as my spirit comes alive, filling my tall broad frame. An Amazon woman.

I realize how much I've been trying to explain my way into feeling or seeming 'normal' despite all the dramatic events in my life that have made me 'different'. Hearing Tenzin speak I suddenly *feel* 'normal', as if there is nothing wrong with me. In fact I feel special, overwhelmingly special. I suddenly feel as though my thoughts, feelings and beliefs have been justified. My whole existence has been justified. I suddenly realize how much immense wisdom I have gained through the hardships I have experienced and I need to acknowledge and value that. With this I feel a huge explosion and letting go of anger, shame, fear and all the feelings that I had to swallow when the people around me had no understanding or compassion of what I was going through.

All the times when the doctors said, "Oh, she's just got anxiety." Well, NO! Maybe I had a serious disease and you didn't know what it was, though I told you over and over that it all started when I was bitten by a tick. Or when I decided enough is enough and I should be treated with respect and I desperately asked for help and the counsellor said, "Oh, just go and have a hot bath and a cup of tea."

My thoughts turn to the people who I thought were close to me who said, "Oh, she's had all these things happen in her life and there's something wrong with her. That's why she's not getting on with us."

Well, NO! Maybe I just didn't want to be your friggin' door mat shit-kicker anymore! And maybe that's why I had anxiety in the first place which led me to be vulnerable to illness. And the cycle goes on and on and on, I realize, until you jump off the un-merry-go-round and stop putting yourself in situations that are not nurturing, and simply love and accept yourself. Even when there is something wrong with you there is actually nothing wrong with you, for beneath all of it our souls are pure. Loving and accepting our self in every cell of our body, to the deepest depths, that is all there is to do.

I bring my awareness back to Tenzin's words where I'm directed into a deep meditation, towards the stillness, silence and spaciousness beyond my physical body. Within, to the core of my being. Very quickly I reach that place of blissful peace and love inside, that beautiful place that I rediscovered all those years ago in my breath sessions guided by Anne.

"Hear the inner silence, feel the inner silence, connect with that inner silence. Gradually be aware of deep inner peace within that inner silence. Rest in that inner sacred space like a child resting in the arms of loving mother ... a child who has lost a mother, who has been longing to find the mother for a long time. Finally the child finds the mother and connects with mother, and finally the child is resting in the arms of the mother. Imagine you are the child. That sacred inner space within you is that mother. Rest. There is no more struggle," Tenzin continues on with a most beautiful meditation.

Sometimes you hear just what you need to hear at just the right moment. This is one of those moments. I feel as though I have been given permission to stay in this heavenly place of deep love, peace and bliss, always. This is where I belong. This is where each one of us belongs. No matter what is happening in our lives, no matter what authority or qualification another holds, no matter how much we love another, we must always demand and give basic respect for another soul. If in any situation you feel that crushing feeling telling you that you are not as worthy or important as another, or maybe you feel more important, take a step back and remember the purity of love within you, within each of us. The purity of our souls. Always value, nurture and treasure your own sacred self within.

17 Some Answers at Last

While blissful feelings of awakening and joy uplift my soul, I am quickly drawn back into the utter devastation and frustration of being stuck in this stupid body with its continued state of ill-health and discomfort. There is something wrong and I have to have some answers. It *must* be Lyme disease and there must be something else I can do about it, I think to myself. I desperately search the internet for more information. According to statistics approximately 300,000 new cases of Lyme disease are diagnosed in the US each year. From one website to the next I find myself staring at the computer screen in disbelief. In horror. This cannot be possible I think to myself as I read, *'Public Health Alert - Biological Warfare experiment on American Citizens Results in Spreading Pandemic.'*

I read more and more stories, more and more evidence, *'Continuing experiments on the public, treatment denial, watching people's symptoms as the disease takes its natural course.'* My head spins. I feel like I'm in one of those sci-fi movies. One of those awful conspiracy films that you watch, but you don't really worry about because you know it's too far-fetched to ever happen for real. But this *is* real. And I am in it! A sickening churning dread fills my stomach. I have to put it out of my mind. I just have to beat this thing!

Online I come across Dr Joseph Mercola, a holistic doctor in America who provides the most up-to-date health information while 'exposing corporate, government and mass media hype which is designed to sell products while taking no real care for people's health'. His partner too has suffered with Lyme disease. Hmm, sounds like my cup of tea. Having just signed up for his newsletter I look in my inbox to see an article about Lyme disease and a link to Dr Deitrich Klinghardt's website who himself suffered from Lyme disease.

I can hardly believe what I'm seeing. Dr Klinghardt is a highly skilled specialist, who is extremely knowledgeable about how to treat Lyme disease and its co-infections naturally and he combines all the mind, body and psychological stuff that I'm in to! All this inner work I've been doing, it's real! And Dr Klinghardt notes the importance of doing so for your physical health! He talks about many co-infections which often accompany Lyme disease which can create severe symptoms affecting every area of the body. Bartonella which can create nervous system problems with pain and buzzing sensations, mood swings, skin, eye, ear, gallbladder and bladder problems, fainting sweating and anxiety. He describes Babesia with the gastroenterological presentation of constant stomach problems, recurring stomach ulcers and/or indigestion being very common. Headaches and neck symptoms, fatigue, sweats, muscle and joint pain, insomnia, depression, anxiety, irregular and pounding heartbeat, air hunger and a feeling of breathlessness that can be due to the autonomic nervous system being affected by Babesia. All of the symptoms I have had are shown to be caused by Lyme and/or a combination of co-infections.

"Thank God! Some answers, *finally!*"

Reading through pages and pages of detailed information and symptoms of Lyme, its co-infections and a very comprehensive treatment plan, everything is finally making sense and looking very hopeful! Dr Klinghardt talks about homeopathics, ozone therapy and treatment similar to the zapping. All these things that are working for me so far. And urine therapy? I guess he means drinking your own. Okay?! Well, despite my aversion I even give that a go. I'm astonished to read that Lyme disease can mimic nearly all diseases and illnesses including autoimmune diseases, Lupus, Multiple sclerosis, Arthritis, Autism, ALS, ADHD, Chronic Fatigue Syndrome, Anxiety, Depression and much more.

In fact Dr Klinghardt says, "We never had in the last five years a single MS patient, a single ALS patient, a single Parkinson's patent who did not test positive for Borrelia Burgdorferi, the bacteria that causes Lyme disease. Not a single one."

He says all insects that bite have the potential to carry and spread the infection. Care should also be taken between sexual partners and it can be passed in the womb to the child. Dr Klinghardt continues on to say that it's very difficult to find anyone who doesn't have the Lyme bacteria present in their system and it's dependent on the healthy function of our immune system whether or not we are affected by the bacteria.

'The healthy function of our immune system.' This I am soon to discover is the most vital clue to all health for each and every one of us. If only I could fast forward time and bring back the knowledge I am to gain over the coming years. If only much of this information was not suppressed by parties with a vested interest. But that is not so, and for now I'm overwhelmed by all the information and treatment possibilities. I realize Dr Klinghardt would have thousands of patients around the world and I doubt would have time to fit me in. I know I won't be going over there. I'm tired of struggling through this on my own. I need support from a practitioner who can work with me one on one.

Quantum Health

I search the internet for homeopathic treatment for Lyme disease. I'm so happy and relieved to find Dr Cindee Gardener, a Molecular Biologist, Homeopath, Herbalist and Nutritional Counsellor who specialises in Lyme. As soon as I read through her site I know she is the one for me. I know with every cell in my body this is exactly what I need! I fill out a twenty-page questionnaire of all past and present symptoms, conditions, treatments and medications. The fact that I became unwell directly after the tick bites and I have nearly every symptom, it is glaringly obvious to this specialist that I have Lyme disease and she gives me a clinical diagnosis. This in itself is a huge relief. To be reassured that it's not just all in my head. I report my experience with the salve and my concerns about cancer and Dr Gardener also adds treatment for this into my protocol.

Contradictory to Dr Klinghardt's views Dr Gardener believes urine therapy could potentially make things worse, so I happily cross that treatment off the list. While I await my homeopathic and herbal remedies I begin having very hot baths each day, inducing a fever as noted by Dr Gardener as an effective tool against Lyme. Feeling like I could pass out easily, I realise this is something that should be done with extreme care and preferably someone with you. It provides enormous relief, so I do it often now. A vision I had many years ago during my breathwork explorations crosses my mind; the method of taking a hot bath and a bottle of Gin to abort an unwanted pregnancy. How ironic. It feels like a strange full circle. Right back to the beginning.

Through online support groups I find myself speaking with hundreds of people in Australia who are seriously ill with Lyme disease, unable to access any treatment or medical support for themselves or their loved ones. It is truly heart-breaking hearing of people, including children and the elderly, struggling and in agony every day just as I have been. Ignored by medical authorities and told to see a psychologist, they are left helplessly desperate for answers and assistance.

My box of herbs, homeopathics and supplements prescribed by Dr Gardener arrives in the mail. Within one short week the adrenalin is not rushing so madly, uninvited through my body as much. The jittery shaky feelings have eased a little, along with the burning in my chest. I still have intense symptoms but any relief feels incredible. So too is the profound relief having professional support after so many years of being fobbed off and told it's all in my mind. I think of all these years struggling by myself while there have been doctors around the world successfully treating people for all the symptoms I've had. Treating them with no need for a positive diagnoses. They are sensible and professional enough to make a clinical diagnoses and provide relief for their patient in doing so. Something Australian medical authorities could be doing for their patients.

An improvement in my condition is perfect timing, for this weekend I'm going camping with my singing group and I'm going to enjoy it! Time to celebrate! It's late in the afternoon at my friends' bush property. I find them down the back outside the stables. Although they're both friendly it seems I've interrupted an argument so I stroll through to pat the horses. I can hear the arguing is becoming very intense, so much so that I feel the urge to wander back out and become a friendly distraction. This does not help. He is now in a rage, a very frightening rage. I see him reach for a gun! In panic I run back into the building and find myself hiding, crouching behind the door in one of the stables. The soft sound of the horse's breath behind me is suddenly muffled by the sound of yelling.

"I've just had enough of it. I'm gonna shoot that bloody horse."

I sink down into the straw as low and out of sight as can be. I hear footsteps coming our way. I close my eyes. Just like when Lily was born, I dig my heels in and go to that place of deep peace within myself. I do not need to let anything outside of me affect me. I hear his angry German voice on the other side of the stable door. A loud gunshot explodes above me.

My eyes jolt open. I look out the window up into the trees above. My gaze follows the curls and contours of the branches of the tall eucalyptus trees. There has been no rain for a long time and all the bark is dry, flaky and peeling away from the trees. The sky is so crisp and blue. What a beautiful day it is out there. What an awful night's sleep. And what a stupid nightmare.

"What was the point of that?" I ask, not really wanting to know and annoyed that such a beautiful morning has begun in this way. I think about poor little Zulu. And what's with the German bloke? I wonder. It crosses my mind that Roderick, my birth father's name, is German. Horses for me represent my free spirit. I guess no doubt my father would have wanted me to die also. Funny that's something I haven't thought about before. Oh well ... whatever ... I'm over it all. I can't be bothered thinking about it.

Camping in the back of my car is not at all comfortable. This weekend of singing is being held at a communal property on the top of a beautiful mountain ridge. Yesterday was a lovely day of workshops, campfires, dancing and feasting. I can't help looking at one of the men on the other side of the room. Why does he look so familiar? I have to keep looking away so it doesn't seem like I'm staring. Gasping aloud I suddenly realize it's Albert! The gunman. Well it's not him but it looks like him. Exactly like him. How curious. I cannot stop staring.

In preparation for our afternoon concert performance the leaders of the group arrange us into suitable positions. Being tall I move to the back. I look at the lady standing beside me and my jaw drops. I look away, and then look back again. She looks identical to my birth mother. Same hair, same glasses, same smile. Even the same teeth! This is sooo bizarre. She looks at me. I smile and pretend to be leisurely looking around the room. My eyes are drawn immediately back to her. Once more I smile and pretend to be glancing at her as I'm looking about the room. Finally I cannot help myself. "I'm sorry but you look so much like someone I know."

"Oh that's okay. You know you are the second or third person who has said that in my life; that I look just like someone. Maybe it's the same person."

"It's my mother actually. My birth mother."

"I have lots of cousins," she says, seemingly excited, "Maybe it's one of them! Ooow, "I'll be your mother," she says putting her arm around me. I laugh and put my arm around her as we sing together. Little does she realize what a profound experience this is. That a complete stranger would give me such a warm and caring gesture. This is quite bizarre. Quite wonderful.

During our lunch break I introduce myself to the Albert look-a-like and his partner. I apologize for staring at him and explain that he looks just like someone I know.

"So who's my doppleganger?" he asks.

"Oh, you don't want to know. Someone I had a lot of trouble with many years ago."

"Well let's hope this is a healing experience meeting me," he says.

"Oh my, it is. I can certainly tell you that."

I look around. We are on top of a hill covered in eucalyptus trees. This place is so similar to our home in Tasmania ... and Albert ... and my mother. I don't know what's happening or what this is all about but I do know it definitely is some sort of energetic healing opportunity. A healing on a very deep level. Dreaming of gunshots and meeting people who resemble those from my past has triggered painful feelings which have been transformed so quickly to be only positive. It almost feels like I'm in some sort of parallel dimension, another world similar to the other, but here I'm understood, cared for and I am safe. A part of me breathes a deep sigh of relief.

As I drive down the long steep and bendy driveway I have a huge smile from ear to ear. I think about the children on this community, many who are home-schooled. They have been running around all weekend, climbing trees, digging in the sand pit, joining in the singing when they feel the urge to do so, then helping their parents sell homemade refreshments during the breaks. I've watched the young ones freely interacting and moving from mother to father, sibling to friend, from stranger to grandmother and grandfather, all the while being nurtured and cared for, included and loved; their input valued and appreciated. With all their needs met, the children are so confident and content. What an ideal beautiful life these children have. It reminds me so much of the life I wanted to create in Tasmania. When I first came here it brought tears to my eyes. This was the sort of life I wanted for my children. While I feel sadness I also feel joy, for this lifestyle and these values *have* been a big part of my children's life and I know it will be within them always.

18 Wise Old Men

After six months on Dr Gardner's treatment plan, she changes my protocol a little. To my dismay I begin to regress. With some trial and error I put it down to the colloidal silver and peppermint oil capsules, which provide relief when I start taking them again. Nonetheless, over the coming months my improvement seems to plateau. I've been shipping the products over from America and eventually decide I must be able to find somewhere here in Australia which provides similar or the same remedies. I search until I find Mullumbimby Herbals. I make an appointment in the hope they can help me more. Jacinta, an amazing earth mother with a huge list of natural health modalities behind her name holds my wrist. Feeling my pulse and looking into my eyes she can tell me almost exactly what is going on within. She tells me my constitution is Vata and I need to be eating warm foods to best nourish my body. This is surprising to me but also a relief. While I've been eating many salads believing it's better for me, I really love warm cooked foods. For the next year or so I see her regularly and receive the most wonderful care and support with Ayurvedic treatment, massage, homeopathics, herbals and any other supplements that test to be supportive to my system. I also carry out tongue cleaning, oil pulling and self-massaging with sesame oil.

With pain and cramping in my back becoming worse, Jacinta's ayurvedic massages give wonderful relief. Detecting many lumps and irregularities in my back and along my spine she shares my concern of the possibility of cancer. I make it clear I have no desire to obtain mainstream testing or treatment and her unwavering support and care is irreplaceable. Peppermint oil as suggested for my spine provides a very surprising amount of relief. Much of the pain and cramping I've been experiencing, while still intense, eases dramatically. Once again I bless the power of essential oils.

Out of the blue a couple of different friends suggest I start a radio show on our local community station. I dismiss them wondering why on earth they are thinking I would be any good at it. Then seeing people struggling with so many conditions and wanting to share all the wonderful natural remedies I'm learning about, I figure I may as well give it a go. I do the training and start a show called, 'The Healing Hour'. I interview many natural and holistic practitioners sharing their work and all the different methods they offer. After fumbling my way into radio broadcasting, I've been surprised how many people tell me I'm a natural. All in the genes I guess.

I attend the screening of a documentary about Lyme disease called 'Under My Skin' in Byron Bay and meet a beautiful, incredible man named John. He and his wife Barbara were both veterinarians with the department of agriculture thirty to forty years ago studying tick-borne illness in cattle. John talks about seeing borrelia bacteria under the microscope with his own eyes and the methods of testing he used so many years ago which are far superior to the flawed methods being used today. Tragically on their own property Barbara and their dog were both bitten by ticks and became unwell. First the dog became disoriented and lost, and later died. Then Barbara became disoriented and very unwell. John recognised this illness as Lyme disease and recalled a bullseye rash on Barbara but to his dismay the doctors would not treat her for the condition. John shares the most horrendous story of suffering, mistreatment and neglect, recounting the drugs, and sixty or so electric shock treatments she received for her mental health condition. He also describes the depression, neurological problems, epilepsy, blackouts and cancer she suffered. Over a number of years and consultation with over one hundred doctors John said only three would listen, one stating that if he treated her for Lyme that would be the end of his career.

John tells me that his wife developed squamous cell carcinoma lesions over much of her body and he believes they were caused by the Lyme disease. When eventually a doctor treated her with antibiotics for a urinary tract infection, for the first time in five years she was able to recognise her daughter again, laughing and smiling. Her skin lesions cleared up and the depression lifted. Unfortunately by this time her health was bad. A tumour in her jaw had returned. Chemotherapy and other treatment was administered. John was worried about the severe herx reactions his wife was having but was refused a referral to another doctor. When she was discharged from hospital after another stay she died later that night. I am totally heartbroken for this lovely, lovely man whose kind heart shines and radiates from his being.

"You need to look into MMS," he tells me. "Jim Humble."

Almost immediately I research MMS. Its healing benefits were discovered by Jim Humble who named it Miracle or Master Mineral Solution. When he was gold prospecting in Africa, two of his men fell extremely ill with malaria. Given some of the solution, they were back up eating their dinner that night and at work the next day. Jim describes his experience going through Africa curing thousands, usually overnight. He was thrown out of one town apparently because the pharmaceutical company told the hospital to get rid of him or they wouldn't stock the hospital. This work became Jim's passion and he has developed protocols for treating nearly every disease, illness and condition. He formed the Genesis II Church of Health and Healing of which he is the archbishop and the protocols are the sacraments of the church. I interview Jim for my radio show and just like John, his warm caring heart shines through with every word he speaks. He explains that as a church they operate under common law and have more protection from the attack of vested interests.

Jim talks about two MMS products, MMS1 and MMS2. For now, I put MMS2 in the too hard basket. MMS1, also called chlorine dioxide/CD ($ClO2$), has commonly been used for water purification for many years. It comes in the form of sodium chlorite ($NaClO2$), one more oxygen molecule than table salt ($NaCl$). Activating it with citric acid or hydrochloric acid (HCl), it then becomes chlorine dioxide ($ClO2$). Similar to ozone but gentler on the body, chlorine dioxide is an oxidiser which is attracted to negatively charged harmful pathogens. It will draw away electrons that hold pathogens together, blasting a hole in them and destroying them, yet will not harm beneficial bacteria which are positively charged. Once this oxidation process has taken place in the body MMS1/CD break down to table salt and neutralised oxygen.

It seems MMS1/CD does almost everything. It kills parasites, viruses, bacteria, and most mould, breaks down biofilm and neutralises heavy metals. That means it should be good against Lyme and any co-infections. As I have discovered, mould can be one of the biggest causes in the breakdown of our immune system creating some very nasty symptoms. Many specialists believe there's no point treating Lyme until we treat mould toxicity. This is also the case with biofilm, a slimy gel-like substance created within our body by Lyme and many other microbes, in which the bacteria live protected from antibiotics and antimicrobial treatments. Breaking down the biofilm is another first step in treating Lyme and many other chronic infections.

I begin taking MMS1. Following directions, I put one drop in a glass and add 5 drops of lemon juice and allow it to activate. It seems to be against everything I believe in to take something that many people say is chlorine and should never be ingested. Sure enough, it soon gives off a very strong smell of chlorine. While I have a small amount of reservation, after looking into the science behind how it works, all my fears are alleviated. I fill the glass with water and drink it. I do this for a few days and notice a very distinct ease in the muscle cramping and feelings of anxiety in my body. It's a huge relief. By the third day I have some diarrhoea. I feel like I'm having a major die off in my head. Not so much painful, as a deep dull ache with extreme brain fog. I also have a lot of tingling and weird stuff all over especially down my right side, often waking feeling partially paralysed and it takes a while to get my right eye working properly. Night sweats come and go along with many strange uncomfortable sensations in my body.

I find a CD (MMS1) protocol by Kerri Rivera, whose son is autistic, and I discover many people with Lyme, cancer and all sorts of illnesses are using the protocol with success, sharing their results in an online support group. I read through and talk with hundreds of people about their experiences, success stories and what to be careful of. Listening to Kerri's talk I start to realise something that seems very strange to me. She says that many children with autism have Lyme disease. I think back to when my symptoms were extreme, when sounds and touch felt like an electric shock going through my body. I realise I had many of the symptoms of an autistic child!

Kerri has a free book available online, *Healing the Symptoms Known as Autism*, with detailed instructions through every step of the protocol; cleansing and detoxing, an intensive parasite protocol, dietary recommendations, replenishing and repairing the body, what to expect, and much more. This protocol seems to cover all aspects of healing on a physical level. Kerri emphasises the need to rid the body of parasites and that it's no point giving too many supplements until addressing parasites which thrive particularly on B12. This she explains is a reason why some people are low on B12 and supplementation will strengthen the parasites. She talks about POWS, or pissed off worm syndrome. When we start taking anything to kill parasites they don't like it and can become aggravated. They may also excrete bacteria and fungus into the gut including A. and G. Haemolytic Strep that causes PANDAS (Paediatric Autoimmune Neuropsychiatric Disorders Associated with Streptococcal Infections) in many children. I'm amazed to hear an infection with strep can cause severe psychiatric disorders which can be treated with CD(MMS1). Kerri also states that often when the parasites are killed, children's seizures stop. This coincides with Dr Clark's findings.

We need minerals especially in any detoxification protocol and Kerri recommends ocean water, the natural minerals of the earth, which we are able to easily absorb. Ocean water contains ninety minerals which is the entire periodic table, revitalizes our cells, and provides conductivity in the brain. Another important part of the protocol is replenishing the good bacteria in the gut. Rose recently gave me some water kefir grains to make fermented drinks for this purpose and it seems to be working really well as I experienced a notable weight gain when I began taking it, which was a huge relief. Kerri goes into great detail explaining every part of this comprehensive protocol. She also regularly updates the protocol with new information and techniques as she finds them. After some time on the CD(MMS1) protocol I am happy with another gain in weight which I presume is due to parasites dying off. For the first time in many years I am no longer struggling desperately to keep weight on. This is an incredible relief.

19 A World Between Worlds

It has been six months since applying the black salve to my back. I've just been for a surf and lifting the board onto the top of the car I feel a sharp tearing sensation in the area of the scar on my back. Immediately I know this is something serious, unlike any back injury I've had before. Over the following months as much as I set positive intentions reaffirming that I am strong, and search for any unresolved emotional issues, I only find the condition of my back on a downhill slide. While it scares me it's nowhere near as bad as dealing with Lyme and those symptoms are improving thank goodness.

Not only being a wonderful sister-in-law, sharing so many wonderful and effective treatments, Rose has become a valued wealth of information. She tells me about her energy healer and chiropractor Andrew who is often referred to as the body whisperer. He works on three people in the room at once. Apparently a correction in one person can spontaneously help another. I wonder how on earth that can be possible. This I have to see! The first two appointments are on my own and provide huge relief. The rest are usually with one or two people. Andrew follows points from my feet, up my legs, then touching a spot on my stomach tells me to breath and stretch open, encouraging me to reconnect to this point in my body where I have become disconnected. Very similar to Geoff the healer in Yamba, he brings his hand into the air as if he's holding something in between his fingers then he quickly throws it away. The difference I feel in my body is incredible.

I often bring Lily to see Andrew since she has so many big wipe-outs challenging the big waves. We are both lying down. Andrew wriggles my feet. One ankle is tight, the other is loose.

"See this?" he says to Lily, as he wriggles my ankles.

"Yes," she says.

I have no idea what he's doing. Nothing wrong with my ankles, but one is definitely very stiff while the other is loose. He moves over to Lily.

"When we release this in you, it will help your mum," he says. Following points along her body he tells her to breath into them.

He returns to wriggle my feet and to our surprise they are now both loose. I lay with my eyes closed, deeply relaxing as Andrew moves from one to the other doing his thing. All of a sudden he and Lily are laughing. I open my eyes so I can look at them to see what's so amusing. I realise my head had been twitching. It seems Andrew had quietly whispered to Lily to watch, then stood above me pulling on points in the air. Each time he did my head twitched up to that side just like a puppet! As usual I'm intensely curious about his seemingly miraculous abilities. Andrew explains that he can see energy, watching it shoot across the room at times. He will touch an area of the body and can hear the frequency of the muscles, detecting any stress or disharmony. Over the following months and years I see Andrew regularly and I have no doubt he has not only helped to improve my overall condition, but he has kept me walking.

Beautiful Byron Bay brings on its charm once again hosting the 'Uplift Festival' where science meets spirituality. My close friends Kim, Jo and I savor the sensory and spiritual delights with workshops, celebrations, music, dancing and beautiful food. A huge lineup of international speakers share a wealth of information and scientific research connecting the psychical and spiritual realms, stories of incredible journeys into the afterlife, deep meditation, poetry, singing and much more, leaving no doubt that the physical and spiritual realm are one. The added benefit of being the host of a radio show is that I have a media pass, giving me unlimited access to the green room! I'm thrilled to be able to speak backstage with such amazing guests as Dr Bruce Lipton, Anita Moorjani, Dr Eben Alexander, Patch Adams and many more.

Bruce Lipton, a cell biologist and one of the first geneticists, bridging the gap between science and spirituality, gives talks on quantum physics and how our feelings and subconscious thoughts and beliefs shape our reality. I'm interested in his thoughts on breathwork, and we discuss these techniques. He also gives me an exercise crossing the arms and legs to activate both hemispheres of the brain and suggests I look into PSYCH-K™. Bruce is just as nice in person as on his videos, like a teddy bear you just want to keep hugging.

Patch Adams must be one of the most deep, thoughtful and considerate people I've ever met. We talk in depth and I find myself sharing some of my own challenges. He supports me in such a beautiful warm and connected way. I feel safe and encouraged to reveal some of my deepest hurt. The depth of understanding he gives me, even for this brief time is an incredible gift of healing. Travelling all over the world, particularly to war-torn areas of poverty, he is a clown who sometimes just sits with people especially the children, to be there for them at the depths of their grief and turmoil. Some of the horrific stories he shares make mine seem so insignificant, but he reminds me that all people's struggles and feelings are significant and some of the poorest people experience some of the greatest connection and love in this world, something the wealthy at times can be missing in their lives.

I'm fascinated by Anita and Eben's near death experiences and the incredible love and beauty they experienced in the afterlife. So much of what they talk about just seem normal to me, much more normal than many things in everyday life. I take home a copy of their books and can't put them down. Eben talks about his adoption, his birth sister who joined him in the afterlife as an angel, and the music which enabled him to move to higher levels of consciousness. He devotes himself to this kind of work now and is co-founder of *Sacred Acoustics*. He gives many talks providing a scientific understanding of brain-mind-consciousness and how tones engender deep transcendental states of awareness. This reminds me of the sound healing Averil has talked about, using the frequency of 432 Hz said to be the natural frequency of the universe, and 528 Hz the frequency of love. Averil and her husband Ian play music with their instruments tuned to these frequencies, just the way Beethoven did. While music during mediation and breathwork has taken me to amazing levels of deep relaxation, I overlooked the powerful benefits of music therapy.

Anita talks about her experience in the afterlife after dying of cancer and her feeling of being a part of everything, being able to sense what other people are feeling, almost being a part of them. I thought that was just normal but now I'm realising maybe it's not the way other people experience life. Suddenly it dawns on me that not everybody feels that way. I've often been confused when I sense things about people and feel a connection with them, when I sense their soul, *feel* their soul and their love, yet their actions and every day feelings are so different. I don't understand why these things I'm feeling and sensing aren't in line with what a person is doing or how they are behaving. Maybe that explains this contradiction I have felt within myself and my relations with other people.

I feel like I want to say to them, "Can't you see?" But then I don't really know what I want them to see, or at least I can't explain it. Maybe because it's not of this realm. I'm beginning to realize I don't need to make others see because as I've discovered everyone is a reflection, in one way or another, of myself. That does not mean accepting another's bad behaviour. It just means letting it go and finding a way to love oneself more as Anita so strongly reveals.

I have a feeling of déjà vu. I'm standing in the garden at three or four years old. Hmm, this is a very significant part of my life but I have no negative memories from this time. No feelings of hurt to heal. No grief to overcome. How very odd. How could that possibly be? I'm in my brother's yard. A place where I spend a lot of time on my own. There are lots of animals, chooks, dogs, birds and sheep, and a big vegetable garden. I love the corn that we grow then smother with butter and salt before eating. When my brother isn't at work I often watch him sculpting or doing his pottery. Piggy banks are his thing. They are everywhere; in the house, the shed and the garden. All different sizes and shapes.

How could I have no negative memories from this time? Not only did I lose my adopted mother, I lost my father for a year also. Dad couldn't cope when he lost his wife, so Shantel and I went to live with Errol, his wife Donna and their one-year old son David. Though I felt a close connection with them, I do remember noticing the bond between David and Donna and feeling jealous of that. I have no memories of grieving though. I have grieved a lot for the loss of my mother during my therapy but I don't remember feeling any grief at that young stage in my life.

Shantel once told me that when our mother first died we were taken to some sort of home while dad sorted things out. Apparently I was crying and crying and she wanted to come to me, but they made her go off to play. It seems that has haunted her for years, possibly all of her life. I wonder after that if I went somewhere else, to a different dimension. Some place where I could feel my mother's love, where I could bathe in it. If I was somewhere in the spiritual realm it wouldn't matter what happened in the physical.

I am in the yard. I'm here often, on my own. It's peaceful. I am peaceful. It feels like the earth, the plants, the animals are my friends, my life, a part of me and I am part of them. We are one. I wonder if I knew my adopted mother was with me. I have known for a long time that she is. Maybe I knew then. Not a conscious knowing. Just a feeling. Like a warm blanket on a cold winter's night.

I think of my birth watching it from the ceiling and it suddenly dawns on me that maybe that was actually a near death experience. Ripped from my mother before she could even see me, before I had a chance to take my first breath. I wonder why that hasn't dawned on me before. Maybe a part of me has never been fully grounded into my body, into this physical world. I see now that I've been in a world between worlds. Not completely in the physical, not completely in the spiritual, yet always feeling like I need to make a choice or learn how to fit into one or the other. But if we are spiritual beings in a physical world, there is no separation.

Di Ellis

It's now been six months since meeting Bruce Lipton and PSYCH-K™ keeps coming to my mind. I figure it's about time to take action on his advice. I go to the PSYCH-K™ website and discover the only course for the rest of the year in my area of the world is commencing this coming weekend, three to four hours drive away. I know I have to do it. I book in and discover to my surprise it's being held in the suburb where I went to kindergarten. Coincidentally it is near to where my birth mother was living when she was pregnant with me. Adding to these strange synchronicities the training is to be held in a convent. A convent!? Of all places to get my hackles up. I later find out that this particular convent was in fact a place where young pregnant women were sent to have their babies to be adopted out.

Churning gut wrenching feelings of grief and suppression fill me at the idea of being in this convent. I know I wasn't born here, but it could possibly be the place where my mother was talked into giving me up. On arrival this deep-seated gut-wrenching feeling is even worse. A feeling I have known many times and accept as a part of my life now. A part that I will always have to work around. During the morning we learn and practise some of the basic PSYCH-K™ techniques and principles, including methods to set positive subconscious thoughts and beliefs, and the trauma release method which is simple yet very effective. We do some exercises similar to what I have seen in the *Brain Gym* for kids which activates both hemispheres of the brain. By lunch time I realise all of the churning in my belly is completely gone. Completely!! I walk to the toilet past all of the rooms that most likely housed hundreds of girls who were forced to give up their babies. Nope, nothing. No more of those horrible feelings consuming my body. Incredible!

After the basic course I follow on with all the higher levels of training and, at the end of the year complete the health and wellness training, happily donning the title of PSYCH-K™ facilitator. I practise holding Skype sessions with one of my fellow students Clare, who helps me to work through more feelings around my mother. I don't know why, but I still have feelings of angst or anger towards her and I don't want to feel this way. We haven't been in touch for a number of years now. I feel fine about that and know I have forgiven her for anything past or present, so I don't know what's going on. With Clare's beautiful soft questioning we discover I'm feeling responsible for my mother's feelings past and present. I set the belief statement, 'I am not responsible for my mother's feelings'. In an instant before even doing the balance process, I feel a huge shift and release in my body and an overwhelming relief. The next day to my enormous surprise I have a message from my mother. I get excited at first, then remember to just meet her halfway. It is a pleasant interaction but goes no further which I am fine with. Everything that Bruce Lipton and Anita Morjani talk about comes to my mind. Once we do the inner work, the outer world will follow.

Over the next year I follow Kerri Rivera's CD (MMS1) protocol finding it more beneficial than everything else I have used. I can feel the chlorine dioxide successfully killing off many pathogens. Balancing the die-off and herxheimer reactions is a challenge. I just want to take very strong amounts and kill it all off but the reactions are too intense to bear, leaving me completely wiped out. Eventually I get to the full dose and continue on at that level. Later I am glad to learn that well respected senior research scientist Dr Stephanie Seneff has researched the mechanisms by which chlorine dioxide works. As well as many other things she is extremely excited to see that it destroys glyphosate and breaks it down to useable compounds in the body. Dr Seneff believes glyphosate is a major contributing factor in autism and discusses the benefits of a maintenance program to protect against toxins. Hearing her words is like music to my ears.

Within Kerri's protocol is also an intensive parasite protocol using two pharmaceutical drugs, Mebendazole and Pyrantel Pamoate to be taken for possibly over eighteen months. I'm reluctant to take unnatural pharmaceutical drugs, so I do some research. To my surprise I discover that Mebendazole, an over the counter worming medication, is well documented for use against cancer! Why on earth is this not common knowledge I wonder? This ties in with a lot of the new research I've been learning about, including the incredible amount of information shared by many doctors from around the world on a docu-series called, 'The Truth About Cancer'. Just as Dr Clark has been saying for many years, it seems parasites, viruses and/or bacteria are the underlying cause of many diseases and illnesses, including cancers. By killing these invaders the cancerous cells can repair or die off. I find a compounding chemist who can provide the correct amount of these two drugs on prescription for an affordable price and I begin the parasite protocol.

While my Lyme symptoms are diminishing, my back is getting worse. One day I bend over to pick a weed out of the garden and feel the tearing sensation in my back again. This time it is worse. My right foot begins to tingle like it never has before. Instinctively I drop to the ground wondering what just happened. I feel my body to see what is going on. I realise this is getting very serious. I slowly make my way to my feet and sit down inside, feeling a little in shock. I run through my mind what must be happening in my body and what I can do about it. I still have no desire to have any harmful invasive testing. Many times I've heard recommendations to avoid a biopsy as it can rupture the tumour and release cancerous cells into surrounding areas and the blood stream. I wonder if that happened when I used the salve. My back was fine for six months after the salve but maybe it released some cancerous cells which have now spread. Great! Just what I need.

I stop surfing for fear of seriously hurting my back and focus more on photography. Every single thing I do now I manoeuvre myself in a way so as not to hurt my back. Sometimes just turning on the shower tap can hurt. I begin to notice as long as I keep my back straight I'm okay. It's the bending or twisting that I simply cannot do at all. Walking down to the beach one day I step down onto a rock, but my foot slips and I land hard on my backside on the rock. Expecting something to break or give way, I sit for a moment in shock waiting to see if I will even be able to walk. To my surprise, I'm fine. I slowly get up and continue on.

I realise that despite the pain and tingling I constantly have, I'm stronger than I thought. My fear eases somewhat. With caution and care, and Lily's help lifting my board in and out of the car, I return to surfing occasionally, only in gentle conditions. One time as I'm paddling back out after catching a wave some whitewash hits me in the face. I feel discomfort in my neck and tingling in my left pointer finger. I softly rub the lump on the left side of the vertebrae in my neck, which I have noticed many times. This scares me, but I keep going. I make a mental note to be more careful when paddling out. I know the full extent of the risks I'm taking but I monitor every wave, checking it won't lead me to a shallow sand bank where my body might be impacted. Riding a longboard I find it easy to get up, but I'm not able to ride my short board anymore. Paddling and standing on the board with a straight back feels perfectly fine and I have no doubt this is strengthening me, helping me to keep going. So is the joy of being in the water.

With determination I compete in the State and Australian longboard titles again. A part of me is saying I am a fool to do this when I'm actually feeling so bad. But there is another part of me that just doesn't want to give up. The conditions are beautiful and not too challenging. No one apart from Lily and a couple of my practitioners have any idea of the intensity of the struggles I quietly face. I really don't need the fear from other people as soon as I mention the word cancer and somehow deep down, I have a

sense that eventually some way or another, all will be fine. No significant placing for me, but just being in the competition is an accomplishment.
Lily on the other hand is surfing very well and makes it through to the final. All of the girls sit in close catching the smaller waves while Lily sits out wide waiting patiently for the bigger bombs. As usual she's last to catch a wave and my nerves are on edge for her. But what a wave! She catches three very big waves. One dredging, dumping wipe-out, and two long rides, all of which evoke excited cheers from the crowd. After her third and best wave I watch her floating around in the whitewash waiting in anticipation for the siren to go off. The placings are called out over the microphone. The commentator announces up to second place and I still haven't heard Lily's name!
I think of how much she has supported me through everything and how brave and strong she has been. I really hope she gets this. It would be such a great reward for her.
"Which means the 2014 Australian longboard junior girls champion is …. Lily Ellis!"
The crowd erupts, cheering and clapping. Her good friends Joel and Declan lift her onto their shoulders and carry her up the beach with the Australian flag wrapped around her. Her face is beaming, smiling from ear to ear, and so is mine. Joel, who Lily has known since she was about one year old, wins the boys title. It was he and his father, in fact, who taught Lily the finer skills of longboarding. His mother and I are good friends and we could not be more proud of them both.
Lily calls some of her close mentors who have played a very caring and influential role in her teenage years to share her achievement. Manso, another surrogate grandfather and president of our longboard club. Daffy who passionately shares the finer art of longboarding with children and adults all over Australia. Bill, our good friend and Lily's big wave mentor who instils a sense of care yet fearlessness when challenging big waves. While I tried for so long to give my girls everything they needed I realise the full depth of the saying 'It takes a village to raise a child' and I'm so very grateful for all the support and comradery we have received.
The friendships we've made keep us going to competitions up and down the East Coast from Noosa to Sydney. We've now found ourselves to be part of a family of surfers from all over Australia. The Noosa Festival of Surfing, one of the biggest surfing events in the world, expands that family introducing us to surfers, filmmakers, photographers and spectators from all over the world. One such highly regarded filmmaker is Californian, Steve Cleveland, who provides tips and encouragement on

my filming explorations. Little do I realise it, but he is later to become one of the strongest supporters of my work as a health advocate.

Volunteering with the disabled surfers regularly, Jemma and Lily love seeing the joy on the surfers' faces just as much as everyone does. I leave the heavy work to the girls now and sometimes wonder if it will be me as a participant rather than a helper one day. I put that fear out of my mind. My main role now is behind the camera capturing their immense joy. I have been to very few events anywhere, that compare to the camaraderie, appreciation, joy and gratitude shown here. This confirms to me that no matter what your level of ability or health, all of us are able to find an activity, hobby or connection with other people which provides a sense of satisfaction, joy and inclusion in life. Ultimately that is what life is all about.

My photography has grown into an immense passion. Each time I follow someone on a wave it almost feels like I'm on the wave with them. I anticipate their next move, watching and learning many techniques. Each good shot that I get fills me with satisfaction, especially when my photos are often featured in the international longboard surfing magazine *Pacific Longboarder*.

Having this hobby is a saving grace, giving me something to enjoy and look forward to, while my back continues to get worse. I'm in constant pain and discomfort. This, along with the remaining persistent Lyme symptoms are a right pain in the arse. Every now and then I wake up gasping for breath, feeling like my heart has just stopped. It's a strange sensation coming from my back through my chest, the areas where I seem to have cancer, almost as if the nerves have short circuited and the message telling my heart to beat has failed. Other nights I awake dripping in sweat, my pyjamas and sheets saturated. Whenever it happens I can't help but think of Bob, the girls surrogate granddad, who told me his wife awoke every night this way due to the leukaemia which took her life. I force those thoughts out of my mind. I don't dare tell him my experience for I know how much he will worry and tell me to see a doctor. But I have seen enough doctors. They couldn't help. I had to find my own way, and that is the way I prefer now.

Seeing Andrew regularly, the relief he provides is enormous. With his extremely gentle techniques I feel a huge release of tension in my body each time I see him and I still have no doubt he is keeping me walking. I realise though, it's time to try the heavy treatment. No, definitely not chemo or any mainstream treatment. Time to give Jim Humble's MMS2 protocol a go. As much as I have faith in Jim, I really didn't think I would go this far. But I have to try. MMS2 is calcium hypochlorite (HOCL). Jim explains that once mixed with water it becomes hypochlorous acid which our own body makes to kill pathogens. Jim suggests that readers do their own research to confirm this, so that is what I do. Sure enough there are many references that calcium hypochlorite becomes hypochlorous acid once mixed with water and there are thousands of medical references to our own body producing hypochlorous acid to kill pathogens.

What is calcium hypochlorite? It's the pool blast you throw into a pool when it has become green and putrid. I was horrified when I first heard this. I know it's not actually chlorine but it seems like it may as well be. Nonetheless I know I need to give it a go. I order the capsules and start the recommended dose. I don't keel over in pain or notice any signs of poisoning. That's a relief! But I do feel all the areas I'm concerned about reacting to this new substance in my body with a lot of twitching and then relaxation in those areas. I take that as a good sign. For the following months I continue taking MMS1 and MMS2 daily and the Lyme symptoms once again diminish, thank goodness!

I find it irritating because I seem to be extremely fatigued while on the MMS, but better to be fatigued than dead. I'm no longer having the adrenalin and cortisol pumping through my body as much as it did previously which is an enormous relief. Any relief is once again blissful. I presume the adrenalin and cortisol was overriding the underlying fatigue that my body was feeling. I did wish for this, for a return to a state of fatigue rather than the horrendous anxiety in my body when those hormones pushed me into overdrive continuously.

As they always were, I notice the chronic fatigue symptoms are worse after exerting myself. But I concentrate on the relief I have gained. I have also observed during my healing journey, a process which seems to move backwards through the stages in which illness developed. With the removal of each layer comes a brief reliving of those symptoms, as I move back through it to my pure self. Despite my improvements I still have a lot of intense symptoms. I realise with each level of improvement just how dire my health situation has been.

Di Ellis

20 Lucky Escape

I come to Byron Bay every week, sometimes twice a week, to see the chiropractor. I often enjoy wandering the streets and shops mingling with and observing the wide variety of people. But today I don't feel well. My back is sore and I'm very irritable. Lily and her friend Caitlin are with me enjoying looking through the shops. There is only so much being inside shops I can do before I become almost claustrophobic and need to get away. And today is even worse so I leave the girls to enjoy themselves and head off to the beach.

I'm angry with my body. Angry at the condition of my health. I've done all the emotional work. I've eaten well for years. This shit shouldn't be happening. I want the good energy that I get from nature to take these stupid shitful feelings away. I drive to a nearby beach and sit in the car for a while looking out at the ocean. The surf is tiny. Barely breaking. Even if there was some surf I wouldn't feel up to going out anyway. Then I see a very large number of dolphins frolicking along the shoreline. Yes! I get changed and paddle Lily's board out into the water. My back is sore, but I don't care. I'm angry with it and I'm over it! I'm friggin' well doing this anyway. I have my camera and I'm sure I'll be able to get some good footage of the dolphins who are often elusive to the camera.

I feel myself slowly become happier and at ease as I paddle in the water. I see the dolphins approach, then they are gone. I look for them and notice they have turned back. They are now moving away. I notice more dolphins at the other end of the beach. I wonder what they're doing and think their behaviour seems a bit strange. I take it as a sign they don't want to be around my angry energy. I don't blame them. I sit near the surfers who are catching the tiny waves in the shallows. It's not long before I notice the dolphins returning. Again I paddle out deeper into their path and wait patiently. A Frenchman swims out near me to observe these beautiful creatures. I film them as they approach, calling and saying hello to the mums with their babies just near us.

"Oh they're beautiful," I say blissfully. "Here come some just here."
"Yes, just here," choruses the Frenchman.
"They're coming under us!" I exclaim as they suddenly approach very fast. In an instant something hits the back of my board and I find myself falling through the centre into the water.

To my astonishment the impact at the back of the board has broken it in half under me. I pull myself onto one half of the board.
"Oh my god, I don't believe it," I say to a man on a stand-up paddle-board I hadn't noticed behind me.
My first thought is that a male dolphin has become territorial. Though I've had a fright I'm not in a huge panic, unlike the poor Frenchman, who is now hightailing it towards the shore.
"There's a small shark here," says the paddleboarder looking around in the water.
Instinctively I pull myself up higher onto the piece of board. Not that it helps with half my body still floating in the water. Nonetheless, I'm able to remain relatively calm. If it was the small shark that hit the board, and if it still wanted to eat me it would have come back to do so, though it might have a sore head now. I realise my camera is still dangling on its string under the water. I pull it up to see if it's still recording. Yep just like all good filmmakers, just keep on rolling! It's comforting when the paddleboarder stays beside me as I flounder back to the beach on half the board, the other half still attached to the leg rope bobbing along behind me. With the waves barely one foot high, other surfers and people on the beach are curious and astounded as I walk out of the water with my board snapped clean in half. Some people think it's a dolphin but most say it must have been a shark. I'm not sure as there are no teeth marks just a big indent and the side fin smashed in where it seems its head has hit the board.
When I meet up with Lily she is in disbelief. Her Australian title board snapped clean in half, but she is more amused than upset. A couple of days later, I show Bill the board and he asks what the teeth marks are. I look in surprise to see four scratch marks on the centre fin. I wonder if it's possible a dolphin could have intentionally or unintentionally done that. I measure the distance between the marks and research dolphin and shark teeth spacing. An exact gap of two centimetres. That means it can't be a dolphin but seems a perfect fit for a small shark. Hmm, okay then, looks like maybe it was a shark. That would explain why the dolphins had turned away and were behaving differently from usual. And possibly, I have to admit that experience may have reflected what I was feeling on the inside. I wonder if this was a bit of wake-up call to snap me out of my self-pity and self-destructive anger. But it's so hard not to feel this way with the continual pain and discomfort in my body.

I look over the footage replaying it many times. I give a journalist friend the breaking story and the local news station ask me to upload the footage so they can use it. This creates a whirlwind of interest in the story with reports in newspapers and media in many parts of the world. Some of the dolphins can be seen clearly in the underwater footage, but only the outline of the creature that hit the board is seen as it approaches. Slowing the footage down I'm quite relieved and thrilled that a couple of dolphins can be seen coming under me into the path of the culprit, making it veer to the side before turning in to hit the back of my board. I wonder, if not for those dolphins what might have happened.

So many people think I should be traumatized because of my ordeal. I try to think maybe I should be, but I'm just not. The board was broken and I had the tiniest little scratch. I know I was lucky to escape with only that. It just feels so insignificant to all that I go through within myself daily. Let's face it I've had so much more pain and suffering from a few tiny little tick bites. I've spent years in agony every single day. Many of those days I wondered if I would make it to the next.

When I go surfing again, I feel fine. I must admit the next time dolphins come near I find myself looking around in the water with a sense of wanting to lift my legs up. It doesn't take long though for me to feel completely at ease with my beautiful friends swimming around me again. I have no doubt that when your time is up, it's up. When it isn't, it just isn't. In fact my trust in the divine timing of the universe and its influence on our lives has become even stronger, enabling me to surrender fully to life's journey.

Once more I found myself unintentionally walking the fine line between life and death. If it's true that we create our own reality why would I create this? Do I have such a strong subconscious desire to escape this life and be in the spirit world? I acknowledge the part of me that was so frustrated that I didn't care about my back. I became self-destructive and a touch reckless in my bid to break free from my suffering. I take this as a message, another push towards becoming grounded and centred, searching even deeper towards peace and harmony within myself.

I know I must use this experience for healing and empowerment rather than another reason or excuse to escape. I remember Mike telling me many times that I was always running away. I got angry at him for saying that. How was I expected to stay in situations that were miserable or terrifying, including living near a drug crazed gunman who was consistently threatening our lives? But after those few little tick bites, I found my life threatened every day from within, with nowhere to escape to. No way of escape. The terror was relentless. So the series of unfortunate events in my life continues. But I have no doubt everything is created from within and maybe, as much as I hate to admit it, just maybe Mike was right.

Di Ellis

21 Sinister Sweetness

During the past couple of years I have watched a number of close friends who have received a diagnosis of cancer undertake mainstream treatment and become sicker than they ever were and soon pass away. There is no way I am going there. I shared as much of my own experience as I could whilst being respectful of their choices. I didn't let them see it, but as each one of them became sick, I was terrified. Terrified of losing my friend as they became weaker and their lifeforce dwindled, but also terrified I would be next. I dug deep, finding the greatest strength within, the deepest trust that I am doing the right thing. Slowly and silently I continued on my path.

One of my friends who passed away was an elderly gentleman. I often went and sat with him and his lovely wife as they shared many of the treatments he had tried, one of them being medicinal cannabis. I was very interested in it myself. This softly spoken little old lady who was supporting her husband made a couple of phone calls. With a few secret code words my parcel was in the mail. We giggled as she cupped her hands to her mouth, "I never thought I'd feel like a drug dealer."

"You are a drug dealer," I teased, and we giggled even more.

I started as recommended with one drop under my tongue. I was worried about becoming stoned so I took it just before bed. I've had enough brain fog to last me a lifetime. The next morning I woke up feeling smashed. Something big had gone on through the night. I could feel it had worked deep into my cells. Every night I took one drop and awoke each morning feeling a little out of it. Some nights I woke up saturated in sweat. The Lyme symptoms seem to have diminished, but not as much as I would have liked.

One day I thought I'd try a drop during the day to see what happens in my body. Around 10 am one morning I took one drop under my tongue. An hour or two passed and nothing much seemed to change. I got on with things and forgot about it. Another hour or so and I began to wonder what was happening. I was feeling dizzy and uncoordinated. I was wondering what was wrong with me. I laughed at myself suddenly realising I was becoming stoned. While many may enjoy the ride I certainly didn't. I spent the whole afternoon completely wasted, my head spinning, eager for the experience to be over. I tried to act as normal as possible in front of Lily with my head in the computer screen pretending to be concentrating hard!

I didn't feel it was having enough positive effect on me to put up with waking up partially stoned every morning but I would like to try cannabis oil containing only CBD, without the THC. CBD short for Cannabidiol, does not contain the psychotropic effects of THC - Tetrahydrocannabinol, both of which are the two most abundant of the many cannabinoids found in cannabis. I know many people have extraordinary success using medical cannabis to treat various conditions including Lyme, cancer, autism, anxiety, seizures, Parkinson's disease and much more, so I look forward to the day this medicine is readily available to those in need.

Over the years I've continued being very active in many support groups for different diseases and illnesses and varying treatment protocols around the globe. To have this direct access to the latest research, studies and experiences from all over the world is an invaluable resource, providing vital information on steps for health recovery. This is a good thing. A very good thing. Yet sometimes what we discover may be shocking and disturbing. I have no doubt that being able to fully surrender and trust in life, trust in the divine, is a vital part of our happy existence here on earth. There are times though when the complete opposite is essential, when everything should be questioned and scrutinized and steps put into place to protect ourselves. And now is one of those times. With this access to information from all over the world I realise the extent to which many effective treatments have not only been ignored, but suppressed.

A report comes out about Dr Bradstreet who was murdered just before he was about to reveal proof that he found vaccinations to be contaminated with nagalase. It seems this doctor had been conducting research when his own son became autistic after a vaccine. Dr Bradstreet is reported to have found nagalase in the vaccines, a protein often made by cancer to stop our immune system from attacking it by targeting the GcMAF in our body. GcMAF is a vitamin D binding protein which activates our macrophages, a type of white blood cells. Without it our immune system is disabled. Dr Bradstreet was using GcMAF in his treatment of over one thousand autistic children.

I think back to when I became sick as a teenager. It suddenly hits me. It was not long after a tetanus vaccine. I am shocked. I share this information in one of my Lyme disease support groups. I hear from many others saying their Lyme came on after a vaccine. A mother then contacts me and says her daughter became unwell after a Gardasil (HPV) vaccine and since tested positive to Lyme and there are hundreds of them. Hundreds of girls with exactly the same symptoms. Exactly the same symptoms I had as a teenager, but much much worse. Not only do they have the nasty array of flu-like and chronic fatigue symptoms, but they are dealing with Lyme as well, many of them crippled. I am shocked at what I'm reading. I contact some of the mothers and talk to them personally. I share widely all the simple remedies that have helped me thus far.

I think back to the information I received when I was pregnant with Jemma suggesting that vaccines were not as safe and effective as thought. I remember Claire telling me that chicken pox often provides a very important developmental step for children, which can promote a growth spurt. And many of the childhood diseases can be good for children to strengthen their immune system. My girls must now have strong immune systems for between them they have had all the childhood illnesses; chicken pox, rubella, measles, whooping cough and mumps.

With only a few blisters, Jemma first had chicken pox when she was one and a half and still breast feeding. As usual I rang Claire for support. She informed me that breast feeding will provide Jemma with my immunity and may prevent a full dose of the illness,. Unless she has a fever she won't have full immunity. Sure enough when she was four many children in our area were being diagnosed and she came down again with only a few spots, but this time a fever. Lily was breast fed at the time so I'm not sure if she has full immunity. Measles gave them both a few days of strong fever and with loving bedrest they got through it fine. Rubella was the same which they caught from children who were fully vaccinated. We all caught whooping cough from a fully vaccinated child and gave it to a fully vaccinated child whose parents thought it was safe to visit despite our warnings. I wish I had known about Dr Suzanne Humphrey's vitamin C protocol which many people report to be very effective. Despite some herbal remedies we were all very sick with the cough lasting for months, nonetheless we got through it. I wish I'd tried homeopathics earlier as that cleared the end of Jemma's cough very quickly. Lily later came down with mumps and looked like a bullfrog with a sore throat for a few days, but otherwise no problem at all.

I continue learning more about the down side of vaccines and continue to be shocked. I do research and discover that millions of Australians and New Zealanders were knowingly given polio vaccines in the early 60's, which were contaminated with the SV40 virus, a cancer-causing monkey virus. The government knew of the contamination but allowed the vaccines to be administered until the next lot of vaccines were available.

This virus has been found in the tumours of grandchildren of those who received the vaccines. I wonder if my grandfather received it.

Again I have to put all of those horrific thoughts out of my mind. I search the internet for information on GcMAF. Websites, articles, scientific literature from all over the world. It seems all tumour cancers including breast, prostate, lung, pancreatic and melanoma are treated successfully. GcMAF has been shown to inhibit angiogenesis, meaning it stops blood supply to tumours, reverts cancer cells into healthy cells, or destroy them. It has also been shown to reduce the metastatic potential of human cancer cells in culture. With the ability to modulate the immune system GcMAF seems to be effective at eliminating or reducing the effects of nearly all diseases and illnesses including chronic inflammation and viral infections, autism, chronic kidney disease, depression, acne, colitis, chronic cirrhosis of the liver, Crohn's, fibromyalgia, hepatitis, herpes, periodontal disease, LMBBS, ME/CFS, osteoporosis, psoriasis and various types of Immune dysfunction including allergies. Research shows GcMAF can halt deterioration in multiple sclerosis (MS), Parkinson's, dementia and ALS, and due to its ability to modulate the immune system it can reverse autoimmune conditions such as lupus and arthritis. It is also shown to be helpful with wound healing and increasing energy production at the mitochondrial level of our cells.

Immediately I know this protein is something I need to get hold of. Clouded by fear and secrecy it's difficult to find where to access this product but I search the internet, ask questions and find a link to a supplier in Bulgaria. It's expensive but I don't care, I need it. My package arrives and I begin taking GcMAF. I notice marked improvements in my symptoms as the cramping in my muscles and anxiety in my body diminish further. I'm absolutely amazed at the incredible difference I feel within my body. Instructions advise to have good levels of Vit D from the sun or a good supplementation of Vit D/K combination. Since we've had cloudy weather I take the Vit D/K drops. A few days later the clouds part and the sun shines brightly, so I bask in its beautiful warm rays.

To my utter astonishment within fifteen to twenty minutes I have a strong but bearable herx reaction. It seems different and not as bad as many of the reactions I've had after some treatments. I find a GcMAF support group where I revel in the sharing of success stories for almost all diseases and illnesses. I hear about a yoghurt called Bravo which allows you to make your own GcMAF and a cream available from France. I purchase the cream and apply a small dab to the lymph nodes as recommended and feel good results. Some people I speak to can't even handle a pin head on the back of the leg because it activates the immune system too fast for their body to be able to cope with and detoxify the die off quickly enough. Every time I'm in the sun now within ten to fifteen minutes I feel my immune system activating, the strange tingling and cramping sensations filling my body. Different to the usual Lyme symptoms. To be honest it seems as though I can feel the macrophages jumping into action and attacking the bacteria and damaged cells. Amazing! I pay my respects to Dr Bradstreet who unwittingly gave his life for this sweet little cream and the amazing benefits of GcMAF to be known to the world.

I've been cautioned that once you start GcMAF you need to be aware that you can become sensitive or even in pain as the immune system is activated and the macrophages begin to attack tumours and any cancerous areas. When this happens those areas break down and need time to repair and rebuild. I'm glad I was warned of this and I'm glad to have some pain in the troublesome area near my liver. Glad because I know it's working. My spine becomes even more delicate and I can feel many areas breaking down. I know this is a powerful healing process and I need to be patient and allow it to occur.

I think back to the ill-health I began to feel after the filling in my tooth many years ago. I'm becoming aware now of the tension, tightness and gripping that has been held within me, within my back for so many years. All this time I was trying to ignore it and manoeuvre my life and way of being around it. I can also see what an amazing job my body has done to isolate the areas of cancer for so long. Though it seems to have spread to many parts of my body, until recently I've been able to function quite well considering. Now I need to be patient and nurturing of my body in this huge process of change, this process of letting go, releasing on a cellular level the old tightness, old beliefs, fears and self-doubts. My whole self is changing. Although my physical structure feels more damaged and broken than ever before, I can feel my spirit strengthening, the phoenix rising within me.

Every year or two I've been holding seminars, sharing the amazing collection of information and techniques I'm learning about, including all of the mind/body healing techniques I've been working with. I invite all my practitioners who are more than happy to come and share their knowledge and wisdom. I thrive on this work and feel it's my calling. During advertising for the seminar I hear from a lady who lives in the area called Diane Sommer. She tells me about her miraculous experience of healing from Lyme disease after having reconnective healing. I'm sceptical, but interested, so we meet.

Quantum Health

Immediately I feel a strong connection with Diane as we share our horrendous experiences bouncing from one doctor to the other with years of chronic and serious illness, being told it's all in our head before eventually receiving a diagnosis of Lyme. After such an incredible improvement in her own health due to Reconnective Healing Diane became a practitioner. As she explains, Reconnective Healing practitioners pay no attention whatsoever to the supposed 'problem' or symptoms. Instead they step in with the consciousness of allowing that person to return to their peak vibration of energy, light and information. This allows for any of the imbalances to simply vibrate out of the picture, as most appropriate for that person to return to their optimal state of health.

Diane now gifts me with some sessions. She holds her hands ten centimetres or so apart with my hand in between. Immediately I feel my hand tingling. She then continues with circular hand motions around the energy field of my body. Over the following week I feel an enormous relaxation of my nervous system. The continual jittery, buzzing sensations pulsing through my nerves which constantly leave me feeling weak, anxious, and vulnerable, have eased dramatically. I'm in awe of the number of amazing healings she performs, many of them from a distance. Walking through the street people call and wave to Di often stopping to speak of the incredible improvements in varying conditions after her healings. She gets me on to tapping again, the emotional freedom technique, which I have used a little in the past and I notice some particular benefits at this time. Becoming good friends we both explore all avenues of natural health and wellbeing sharing the results of the new treatments, remedies and healing methods we discover with each other and anyone else who might be interested.

I feel more improvement again when taking steps to counter electromagnetic radiation. I buy a Tesla Bluesheild device after attending a talk given by Donna Fisher at a cancer seminar. Designed to emit healthy frequencies which our body resonates with, the device neutralises the effect of the negative EMFs. I buy the personal device and again I feel a very definite settling and strengthening of my entire nervous system. I also have a Geocleanse orgone negative ion generator which is plugged into a power point in your home. This was another recommendation from Rose who noticed a big difference to her health and her nervous system as soon as she plugged it in.

Curious, I go looking for more information about orgone or orgonite. I come across information about chemtrails with aluminium, barium, strontium and some sort of fibres, but I put that in the too hard basket and focus my attention back onto the orgonite. Coined by Austrian scientist, philosopher and psychoanalyst Dr Wilhelm Reich in the first half of the twentieth century, orgone energy is bio-energy or universal life force energy also known as chi or prana. During his research Dr Reich discovered that organic materials attract and hold orgone energy, while non-organic metals simultaneously attract and repel the energy. Orgonite is created by combining resin, classed as organic, and metal shavings, classed as inorganic. Quartz crystal is added to this mixture due to its piezoelectric properties when under pressure, such as the constant pressure when resin shrinks, quartz gives off a charge. As a result, negative energy, which is constantly attracted and repelled in a 'scrubbing' action is cleansed leaving healthy orgone energy. While some claim this is based on pseudo-science many people report positive effects when using orgonite, such as a sense of calm and relief of symptoms related to exposure to electromagnetic radiation. Coincidently I meet a local man who makes orgonite and I buy some necklaces for myself and my girls. With an intriguing story he talks about clearing the sky with 44 gallon drum sized orgonite, and microwaves used as electronic harassment and mind control. I come to the conclusion some stories are best left untold.

22 Positive Results

I'm sitting in circle with a beautiful group of women. We share, laugh and support each other to the depths of our souls. We openly commit to honouring and holding space for the strongest and most sensitive parts of ourselves. Sharing anything and everything which contributes to the enhancement of the physical, emotional or spiritual aspects of our lives, we have a deep respect for each other. A new member to the group tonight is lovely Isabella. In conversation at the end of the evening she tells me about a strange sounding plasma energy device, called a Theraphi. I'm offered a free trial session which I'm delighted to accept.

Arriving at the clinic I meet her work partner John with whom I feel an instant affinity, as I did Isabella. After a short conversation I know these are two people I can trust with my deepest darkest and most sensitive feelings. When I walk into the session room I spontaneously take a step back and ask if the effects would be lingering from the last session. I feel almost as if I've walked into a new energy field. I'm told it's quite possible. There are two glass tubes perched on stands with wires leading into a device. I sit down in between the two tubes and I'm given a cushion to sit on, lifting me a little higher so the troublesome area of my back is directly in line with the tubes. John switches the Theraphi on and the tubes light up, glowing a luminous pink.

I feel a sensation of pressure on the inside of my back at the area of the scar, which builds very quickly. The pressure becomes so strong I feel like I might have to jump up out of the field. But I stay and soon the pressure remains strong without building any more. I can feel precisely the area being affected which gives me a visual image of a tumour or mass of damaged cells on the inside of the scar going down towards the lump in my abdomen, which is also feeling the pressure. Almost immediately after the session the cramping down my right side has eased dramatically. During the next week I have two sessions a day. Each time, I feel it working in damaged areas. As one area eases the pressure builds in another. It feels like it's working on the area that needs it the most first, before moving to the next area of priority. I don't know exactly what it's doing, but again I feel a strong sense of letting go and breaking down of these 'stuck' damaged areas of my body and I have an improvement in my overall condition.

I continue with all my potions rubbing the GcMAF cream down my spine and taking the MMS1/CD and MMS2 depending on what feels right at the time. I also incorporate one of Jim Humble's protocols which uses dimethyl sulfoxide, also called DMSO. This organic sulphur compound is a by-product of the paper making process and was discovered in Germany in the late 19th century. This doesn't sound so good but it seems well known for it's healing properties. A colorless liquid, it has gained notoriety for its ability to penetrate skin and other biological membranes and has been used at times to increase the body's absorption of other medications. DMSO itself is reported to have potential clinical applications in the treatment of a number of conditions such as depression, fibromyalgia, arthritis, interstitial cystitis, athletic injuries, congestive heart failure, diabetes, cancer, AIDS and Alzheimer's.

Following Jim's directions I activate a large amount of MMS1/CD wait a minute or two and then add the DMSO, which is meant to draw the MMS1/CD through the skin and into the cells. I apply this solution to different parts of my body throughout the day as directed and continue each day after. Within a day or so I notice a big difference. My breasts become tender as does my spine. This is a good sign to me. I know it's working. On one of the support groups I also hear about *The Perfect Storm Protocol* for cancer which is almost identical to Jim's DMSO protocol. Coincidentally they talk of a plasma device similar to the one I've had treatment with, which is used with this protocol but not essential. They also recommend the same liver flush process that Dr Clark uses. Talking with people in the support groups it is reassuring to see the success people are having with such affordable treatments.

One of my holistic doctors introduces me to German New Medicine which has shown mapped areas of trauma in the brain which perfectly correspond to areas of cancer in the body of hundreds of patients. I remember Averil talking about this powerful form of medicine which she has used during her journey of healing after being diagnosed with multiple sclerosis due to a hep B vaccine. Within a week of her first shot she was paralysed from the waist down. She recovered and without realising the cause of her condition went for the second shot and the same thing happened; paralysis from the waist down again. She was later diagnosed with MS which was proven in worker's compensation court to be a result of the vaccine. She refused advice from specialists that she would most likely be in a wheelchair within six months and has spent twenty years active and well thanks to the brilliant work of holistic doctors and specialists, and her commitment to exploring many forms of healing for mind, body and soul. Averil has put me onto so many seemingly weird and wacky treatment options, which when you look into the science behind how they work they aren't actually weird at all. They are common sense techniques discovered by very intelligent free-thinking researchers.

My doctor also introduced me to biochemistry and I had the pleasure of meeting Dr William Walsh, author of *Nutrient Power*. He has developed natural treatment protocols used by doctors throughout the world for patients with behaviour disorders, ADD, ADHD, autism, depression, anxiety, bipolar, schizophrenia, Alzheimer's Disease and more. With a scientific database of 25,000 patients and a million assays of chemical factors in blood, urine and tissue, Dr Walsh can look at someone's blood chemistry and accurately predict which mental health condition they have.

Dr Walsh shared his knowledge of thirty plus years' research experience at an annual conference held by Bio-Balance Health. Doctors come from all over the country to train in these methods. This not for profit organisation, was initiated by two Australians in 1998. They were so impressed with the work being done by Dr Walsh and his colleagues in treating patients with mental and behavioural disorders, using simple natural supplementation to correct their biochemistry. They resolved to take action to make these assessment and treatment techniques available in Australia. I have heard many of the conditions Dr Walsh talked about mentioned in the Lyme disease support groups such as MTHFR gene mutation, over and under methylation, and pyrrole disorder. He also talked about copper overload, zinc deficiency and heavy metal toxicity having a huge effect on health, particularly mental health.

I also listen to the Anxiety Summit hosted by Trudy Scott who explains some of these conditions in more detail. She also talks about simple amino acids that have the potential to completely alleviate anxiety and depression. If you are lacking the amino acid Gaba it could be the cause of physical anxiety in the body. If it is the cause of your anxiety, relief can be felt within five minutes of supplementation. If you are lacking the amino acid L-Tryptophan you may have depressive or anxious thoughts. I immediately order both of these supplements to give them a go. Trudy mentions if you have sleep issues or high cortisol, tryptophan is helpful. She describes many other simple supplements which can be very helpful for many conditions and types of anxiety and depression and suggests to work with a qualified practitioner for best results.

I have some testing for these conditions. Pyrrole disorder and zinc deficiency show up, one MTHFR mutation and some hormonal imbalance. Zinc supplementation makes me feel a little ill, but when I receive the compounded pyrrole mixture containing zinc, magnesium, vitamin E and B6, I tolerate that much better and feel a very strong activation of my immune system.

Another intense activation of my immune system occurs when I begin making my own GcMAF with milk kefir. My supply of GcMAF cream has been cut, the producer accused of making false accusations regarding the effectiveness of the cream despite hundreds of people I've spoken to sharing their successes with all sorts of differing conditions and illnesses. I heard about making your own GcMAF a long time ago and look for information and recipes. Though most recipes include specific bacterial strains which you need to buy regularly, I decide to have a go without them. I buy some milk kefir grains from my local health food shop, some colostrum which contains the GcMAF and some organic raw milk. I combine all ingredients in a jar and within a day or so I have my own concoction ready to try. The next morning I awake to my spine, hands and feet tingling like crazy. I lie still wondering what the heck is happening. I try to work out how I could have hurt myself or what may have happened during the night to cause this.

I suddenly realise the GcMAF produced by my milk kefir must be very strong and has activated my immune system to attack the damaged areas in my back. This feels just like when using the GcMAF drops and cream but even stronger. Again it seems like I can feel the macrophages doing what they are reported to do - engulfing and digesting cellular debris, microbes and cancer cells, and anything that is not conducive to a healthy body. Through trial and error I work out a good amount for me to take so as not to activate my immune system too much. I give myself breaks allowing my body to recover and strengthen each time after damaged areas are broken down. I'm finally beginning to learn slowly, slowly. I don't need to be in a panic. It took years for this state of chronic dis-ease to develop in my body. I accept, as much as I can, that it will take time to reverse this process.

Week after week, month after month I feel myself improving. I usually spend from daylight to dark on the computer researching topics and learning more from other patients, doctors and scientists and supporting other people sharing all that I've learnt. Since I haven't had intensive testing or a biopsy I'm frustrated that I can't really say with conviction what is happening in my body. If this is a process of recovery from a serious case of cancer, I would like to have some evidence. Then I would be able to share more openly with people, but as it is I presume many would think I'm imagining the severity of the problem. I talk to one of my doctors about having an MRI. He asks me why I would want to expose myself to the risks of such testing especially when my whole system has been so sensitive. Instead he recommends thermal imaging as a safe option. With further research and after speaking to Lyme patients who have had very bad reactions from MRI testing I am relieved I didn't take that step. I decide to get some thermal imaging in the hope of having some evidence of what has been happening in my body before it's completely healed.

I search and find Gold Coast Thermal Imaging, and with anticipation go for an appointment. I explain to Nicola, the technician, that I'm actually really hopeful of finding something. Talking about my situation she's very interested in all the different treatments I've used and their results. Having her own experience of holistic healing Nicola is extremely knowledgeable. I fill out the forms including a detailed drawing of the areas which I believe are affected. I explain that it's mainly in the areas where there seems to be cancer, that I feel the Lyme symptoms now and as I improve those areas are becoming less. Holding my arms above my head I'm directed to stand in certain positions for the camera. I'm asked whether I've had any problems with my breasts, any swelling or lumps at all, and I reply that I don't. Only a bit in the past, but nothing I've been concerned about.

Most people would be horrified but I'm delighted when abnormalities show up in almost exactly the areas that I drew. My neck, shoulders, spine and areas of my abdomen, particularly the right side around the liver. With most of the abnormalities showing up on the right side it's very clear the problem has originated from the hidden tooth abscess. Fantastic! More proof that it's not all in my head! To my surprise, abnormalities also show up in both breasts, hence the questioning. After dealing with Lyme and what looks like cancer of the spine, learning that it seems to also be in my breasts just doesn't even register any concern. I'm so much better than I was and I know I will only continue to improve. Nicola sends me information regarding oestrogen dominance and its connection to some cancers, and links to experts such as Dr Christiane Northrup and Dr John Lee.

During the past year or so, a senate enquiry into Lyme-like illness in Australia has been underway. Having attended the Brisbane and Sydney hearings it was heartening to meet such caring and understanding senators who are determined to have proper recognition, diagnoses and treatment of Lyme disease, or Lyme-like illness in Australia. Evidence shows Australia does have one or more forms of Borrelia bacteria which could possibly cause all of the symptoms of Lyme, but there is heated debate about whether Borrelia Burgdorferi the specific bacteria which is linked to classic Lyme disease is here.

Representatives from health departments argue they have been unable to confirm Borrelia Burgdorferi in Australia. With persistent questioning from one of the senators, who is becoming very frustrated with the ignorance that is being displayed, they are forced to admit the testing methods in Australia are outdated. All of the people in attendance are horrified to hear such lack of professionalism regarding such a serious issue. Patients like myself don't care which bacteria it is or what it's called. Many of us know we were bitten by ticks and have many, if not all of the classic Lyme symptoms. We just want proper support and treatment. Jenny Bourke, an independent Australian pathologist confirms that their internationally accredited laboratory has detected Borrelia Burgdorferi for many years in patients who have never left Australia.

The senators meet with and listen to hundreds of patients across Australia, local and international doctors, researchers and specialists; resulting is a senate report tabled in parliament which recommends that, *federal, state and territory health agencies, through the Council of Australian Governments Health Council, develop a consistent, national approach to addressing tick-borne illness. As a matter of urgency, they are to develop a cooperative framework which can accommodate patient and medical needs with the objective of establishing a multidisciplinary approach to addressing tick-borne illness across all jurisdictions.*

There is much excitement with the release of this report which soon turns to bitter disappointment. While some committees and meetings are set up no action is taken by health authorities to actually address the problems. In fact two weeks later I attend a suicide prevention meeting and two local doctors inform me they have received notice that there is no Lyme disease in Australia. No talk of addressing tick borne illness at all. I am devastated and disgusted. I knew there was something seriously wrong with our medical system, but I didn't realise it was this bad. The only thing I can do is continue empowering myself and others. Through Jenny's lab Australian Biologics, I have testing for Lyme and finally receive a positive diagnosis for Borrelia Burgdorferi confirming what I have known right from the beginning. I work hard to transform my anger and frustration at health authorities into positive steps I can take to support others and share beneficial information.

Through the online support groups I hear about the benefits of bicarb of soda, something I heard about briefly many years ago for cancer treatment. I attend a talk put on by a company called Safesoda and I'm enthralled with the information provided in this fascinating talk. They mention that a man's pH level was so low they didn't know how he was still alive. Immediately I start the protocol and test my saliva pH level the next morning. Sure enough, no surprise, it's the lowest it can be. Within minutes of taking the bicarb I have complete relief of remaining Lyme symptoms. The cramping, tingling and tightness in the muscles along my spine and neck, tingling in my tongue, the breathlessness, and the underlying feeling of anxiety in my body, all completely and totally disappear! I can't believe it.

I take one teaspoon four times a day as recommended. Over the next few days all the areas that showed up in the thermal imaging are aching especially my right shoulder, all the way through on the inside and high on my right breast. I am amazed! I can feel all down my right side being affected, the areas where the poisons from my tooth would have drained down into my body. I remember going water skiing many years ago and all the muscles I would normally not use ached like mad afterwards. This is how I feel now. Like all these muscles are opening up, activating and repairing. Dean said that many people with arthritis can have pain as the arthritis breaks down when taking the bicarb. I'm sure it's the breaking down and regenerating process that is happening within me now. I find the bicarb is so effective at relieving all of my symptoms I don't bother taking anything else for the next six months. This is incredible. All those years ago when I heard about the benefits of bicarb. It seems this simple and cheap remedy could have alleviated all that agony.

I look back to when I was in hospital dying, being sent home and told I had anxiety. I hold no resentment. Well, hmm, no point kidding myself I guess. I'll work on that, but I'm so glad I was sent home without being given any invasive treatment. There is no way my body would have handled anything else, and I know I would be dead now. Actually, come to think of it, I'm not glad that happened. It just shows the complete failure of our medical system to treat chronic health conditions. I imagine what it would be like if our hospitals provided a diet of nutrition and simple cleansing, holistic and integrative therapies. So much suffering could be alleviated. So many people could recover their health. This would relieve the hospitals of overcrowding, enabling them to do the brilliant work they excel in during acute and serious situations. I wonder what my life may have been like if that were the case years ago? How my health would be. And if many of the simple time-tested remedies I've used were readily available back then and my adopted mother and step mother had access to them? What a different world it would be. What a different life I would have.

23 Reflections

One of my first memories at three and a half years old is at the hospital before my adopted mother died. When I was pregnant with Jemma and having counselling it was suggested to draw any pictures or images that come to mind. There was one strong image I drew. I asked Dad if it made any sense. He looked it over.
"It was Christmas Day. We were at the hospital visiting your mother. She was in an isolated room. Facing out to the garden there," Dad says, pointing to the picture, his eyes tearing up. "That would be you and your sister when the doctor took me aside."
I look at the drawing in my hand. My sister Shantel and I are standing at the large window looking in at our mother lying on a bed. I listen as Dad weeps, explaining that was when the doctor told him she was going to die. Three weeks later she died from hepatitis. They hadn't known what was wrong with her for quite some time. A very conservative stay at home mother, I guess they didn't suspect hepatitis and they didn't know where she acquired it. One day I was looking at an old photo of me when I was maybe a year old. I don't know why but I opened the frame and to my surprise behind the photo I found an envelope addressed to my mother which had been posted by her sister. Inside was a newspaper clipping about a rabbit plague on the Nullarbor. I have no idea why this clipping was in the frame, or who put it there. I can only guess it was my mother. Nor do I know why I carried that photo in its frame around with me for years while I have no others.
It's quite ironic that I too nearly died due to a problem with my liver. If my mother was given something so simple as alfalfa leaf tea to cleanse her liver I wonder what the outcome would have been. Looking back I can see clearly the enormous amount of tension that I've held in my body for most of my life. I did not want to feel, so I held my feelings down. I created a life on the outside that was good, but I did not want to feel how I felt on the inside. Feeling was too painful. I actually remember thinking to myself that even if there was something wrong in my organs I just didn't want to know about it; it would be too hard to deal with. Yet it was holding my feelings down, holding the tension in my body, which inhibited my organs and my whole system from functioning properly and contributed to my illness, recreating that same pain all over again.
All those years ago the counsellor recommended Louise Hay's book and it's been a constant go to in my life. I follow her principles of healing daily,

always looking for the emotional connection to any physical problem. I can reference her book in my mind now, but often I find my own answers. I ask a question and the answer usually comes to me. As I question and re-question myself I continually look for ways to improve my patterns of thinking, replacing negative thoughts and feelings with positive affirmations.

I have learnt that you *never* need to go looking in the past for problems. There are always problems that can be found if you want to look for them, but by doing so you may be recreating and reliving pain which may well have been better left in the past. When you live in the present moment and move *forward,* towards the life that you want to live, any problems that may need to be addressed will effortlessly present themselves if you allow them. There may be some parts of yourself that simply cannot be healed, some wounds that are just too deep, but you can find a place within yourself that is untouched, a part of you that is pure and can never be hurt. When you live from that place there is no pain. You don't need to get rid of the other parts of yourself. Nor do you need to fix them. Just accept them and love them.

Though I have always felt very strong in who I am and how I want to be, I have at times felt very confused about where I fit in. I was a firstborn, yet grew up as the youngest of eight. A number of my adopted siblings, who were the same age or older than my birth mother, were more like aunties and uncles. Each has had an important impact on my life in their own way. As we grow older I'm beginning to feel a little more like a sister than a niece. I guess it might explain why I have often found myself enjoying the company of people a little older than myself. With the combination of my adopted and step family I've had so many varied and wonderful people as role models and influential figures in my life. I have felt and experienced the love and good in all these people. At times, with many different or opposing beliefs and values, I have felt torn between one way of life or the other. With so many opposing sides to myself, I often felt like I had a split personality. But I learned to accept those different sides of myself, thriving on a wide range of experiences and influences.

When I became a mother I wanted to free myself from any and all negative patterns I had inherited. Little did I realise what that would mean. Even though it has been an enormous challenge, I would rather have those challenges, as well as all of the love that has been in my life, than to be without either. For years I've observed the patterns, differences and similarities between myself and my adopted family, my birth family and my step family. When I was born, my birth mother was eighteen and she had been training as a nurse. Her mother, who wanted to raise me was close to fifty. When I was adopted I had a sister who was eighteen and was training as a nurse. Interestingly our mother also was close to fifty. Strangely, my sister and my birth mother both married men with the same name.

I have had the unique opportunity to be my own case study, exploring genetic influences compared to environmental dynamics. At times my adopted father and I had the same symptoms for totally separate reasons. It was a number of years ago, following a hip operation, Dad told me that he was experiencing trouble in his right shoulder and arm with numbness and tingling along the outside of his right hand and small finger. I was astonished, for at the same time I too was having exactly the same trouble in my right shoulder and arm and tingling in my right hand and small finger. I didn't know then what was causing my affliction but I certainly do now.

I've had two fathers. One who I've never met. The other, my rock, there for me always despite any problems, to help me in any way he could. I have inherited traits from them both. Whilst I'm a very committed and reliable person, I also do not like to be tied down. Many times I've felt torn between those two urges. To be stable and grounded, or to be free and wild. Now I have discovered that the more freedom and expression I allow my emotions, my thoughts and my creative desires, the more stable and grounded I am. I realise that unsettled rebellious part of myself was in some way a part of me that knew something was not right. That a part of myself that was desperately needing recognition, acceptance and expression so I could truly thrive. If we try to conform too much to other people's or our own expectations we can suppress a part of our spirit, a part of our lifeforce. On the other hand if we are not grounded and practical our creative potential may never manifest into reality. It is important for each of us to find a healthy balance in our own lives.

Having had three mothers each playing an equally significant role in my life has also provided confusion. I've had one mother who gave me away, one mother who died and another who was mentally ill. During my ill-health and long healing process I've had times when I just wanted to die. But I knew I couldn't. I knew what it felt like to lose your mother, so I had to keep going for my children. I had to find a way to get better whatever it took. I have had occasions when I found it so difficult being a mother that I felt as though I could just leave. But I couldn't do that either. I knew what that felt like. Working through muddled thoughts, dreams, nightmares and grief there were so many times it all felt too hard. I just wanted to give up and allow myself to go insane so I didn't have to care or think about any of it. Yet I knew what it was like to have a mother whose spirit was gone, leaving at times an empty shell of a body. That too was not an option. I felt trapped emotionally, physically and spiritually. Trapped within myself, with no escape.

The only option was to find a way to deal with it all. After slowly working through those gut-wrenching feelings of grief, abandonment and loss, I found I was able to see and feel the incredible amount of love that each one of my mothers gave in their own way; each one giving me a form of emotional, physical or spiritual love that the other may not have had the strength or ability to give. I began to see and feel the incredible amount of love in myself and this world. Now I thank God I was trapped. I thank God I did work through all those feelings. I thank God I am able to enjoy the love that I feel within and share it with the world around me.

My message to you is that no matter what is happening in your life try to find, within yourself, that part of you that is untouched, pure, always loved and strong. Your soul, your spirit. The parts of you which are eternal. From this place anything and everything is possible.

I have learnt that your deepest heartfelt love within can never be taken away by anyone. If you love someone deeply, be they a partner, friend or family member, even if they do not reciprocate in the same way, your own feelings of love remain. They're a special part of you to keep and to hold onto, if you wish. Your life may need to go in a different direction from that person but that love within need not be taken from you. This awareness has given me the ability to open my heart fully. To relax and let go of the fear of hurt from relationships and the corresponding tension this creates in the body.

While it is a blessing to be able to learn and widen our knowledge, health isn't so much about *knowing*, it is about *feeling*. Allowing ourselves to feel all the feelings that we have, such as happiness, anger, fear, sadness, joy and most of all love. Though we may need to respond to certain situations and make changes, sometimes the most important thing we can do is to manage the way we respond and bring our awareness to our body and our feelings, allowing ourselves to feel the full depth of them. By doing so we are allowing the energy in our body to move. Just as Bruce Lipton and many amazing scientists and researchers have found, our emotions actually are 'energy in motion'.

Letting go of the outcome of a relationship can be the hardest thing we ever do. Whether it be a child, parent, partner, sibling, other family member, or a friend, we are deeply connected on an energetic level to the people we are close to. This letting go does not necessarily mean letting go of the person. It may do. But letting go means letting go of any expectations for that person to make us feel good. Instead we need to go within to release anything which is stopping us from feeling good from the inside. Doing this we allow the infinite love and joy from within us to spontaneously arise, to be shared with our loved ones and everyone around us. This in turn will attract deeper understanding and love into our lives. At the same time holding on to the people we love, showing them how important they are in our lives, creates the structure, strength and foundation of our life.

Di Ellis

24 Back to Where it All Began

"You have to come and visit this year before I move back to Oz!" Nikki insists.
For twenty years she's been asking me to visit her in New Zealand and now I just have to do it! I plan the trip with my girls so we can see my sister Judith and go to a surf competition while we're there. I might even put my feelers out for my birth father and possibly connect with my Uncle who I've never met.
We're at the airport with our close friends Corey, Yasmin and their children Jay and Tawny, another surfing family who are joining us on the trip. Warnings have been out for a couple of days and Cyclone Debbie is now playing havoc. One may have taken this as an omen for the rest of our trip, but really what is one to do? With flooding, torrential rain and gale force winds domestic flights are cancelled but our international flight goes ahead, much to Yamin's dismay as the plane drops and jolts through the intense turbulence. Lost boards, flat phones and lost accommodation at 3 am. The next day running around looking for boards, getting them through customs, a large currency conversion, and a speeding ticket for my first drive in NZ. What a start to our trip! Pulled over by police with blue lights and a siren captured on video, combined with some good acting turns into a serious April fool's day joke, al la Lily! The joke works very well when she seemingly arrives home in the middle of the night on her own in a panic, but it goes bad as Corey and Yas equally in a panic, ring the police wondering how I could have been arrested for stealing money from some strange man lingering at the currency exchange. As I make my midnight entrance Corey clues on to the fact that we are now into the wee hours of the first day of April. With frustrated and amused laughs all round we breathe a sigh of relief.
The next morning we arrive at the beach in Sumner, Christchurch, the sun rising and small waves peeling perfectly into the bay for *The Single Fin Mingle,* an international competition. The surf and the vibe are simply divine. The sweet sounds of jazz music float through the air. Gentlemen young and old don moustaches, berets and tweeds while the ladies parade their vintage retro dresses. One would think one was actually back in time or on the set of a movie. A photographer's dream, the surfers catch wave after wave under the tall cliffs, passing a quaint little white and blue boat house, the perfect backdrop. For three days we have been warmly welcomed and entertained, but now, with a traditional Maori

ceremony bidding us farewell and a safe journey, it's time for our next adventure.
We head to the beautiful coastal town of Kaikoura, known for its abundance of seafood and a long right-hand point break. Unfortunately there's not much surf but Corey, Jay, Jemma and Lily go anyway catching a few waves. Seven people, six surfboards and loads of luggage all squashed into the ten seater Usave van with Corey at the wheel brings constant entertainment. The joy and laughter on this trip is not quite, but almost equalled by the bickering and arguing when two families are cramped for too long in small spaces, each family seemingly taking turns quarrelling to the amusement of the other. All that keeps coming to mind is National Lampoon's Vacation! Rain and new slips prevent the earthquake damaged coastal road back to Christchurch from opening at 7 am as expected. As we wait in the line-up of cars the minutes turn into hours and the Usave becomes a hotbox of tension. We'd much rather be sitting in a line-up of surfers.
"Argh, National Lampoon's Vacation!" I proclaim with a laugh again. When the road finally opens at 9.20 anxiety turns to relief. That is until we realise only one lane is open all the way, with traffic controllers guiding us precariously through the damage and road works. The mountains meet the sea with rugged coastline to our left and sheer exposed cliffs to the right. Nervously we peer up, watching small rocks and debris cascading down the broken hillside to the road. Shipping containers held by cables bolted into the hillside are lined up ready to catch the larger rocks. Some are caved in due to the car sized boulders which have come thundering down. An impatient drive along this spectacular route to reach the airport by the 12.30 pm bag drop ensues, nonetheless we give up on worrying about missing the plane and enjoy the windy, misty ride.
Enthralled and distracted by our drive we have forgotten to organise our belongings. 12.17 pm the Usave screeches into the airport drop off and a cascade of people, bags, boards, food, water, rubbish bags, wet towels and wetsuits fill the footpath, onlookers staring in disbelief.
"If I miss the plane I'll be on the next one," yells Corey as he takes off to return the Usave.
"Let's go, let's go!" I yell to everyone.
Our luggage is checked in very late. "They'll come on the next flight" the assistant tells us. "Just run!"
Somehow at 12.57 pm we all sit down in our seats and the plane heads for the runway. The smiles turn to laughter and all feelings of angst

dissolve into a huge sense of accomplishment. Landing in Auckland we fly straight into cyclone Debbie once again, which has made its way across the Tasman Sea. There are weather and flood warnings for many areas. Really?

In a little old three seater van the girls and I travel north. We laugh at Corey and crew who wait two hours and still don't have their plush fancy van. We've barely driven ten minutes before the rain and wind halt us to a slow crawl on the highway. We receive photos from our travelling companions eating from their complimentary five star accommodation and seafood buffet, put on by their van company who were unable to provide the vehicle until the next day. We return photos of our dinner; dry biscuits provided by the fellow Aussie travellers in the lane next. This was highly amusing for all of us. For me, every moment just living, breathing and enjoying life is awesome.

The girls and I receive an abundance of love and nurturing from my adopted-sister Judith and her husband Kevin who have prepared some delicious home cooked goodies. Though I've only seen Judith every now and then over the years, my connection with her has always felt strong. I guess our bond developed during those first three years of my life. She tells me how much she loves me and always wished she had kept me when our mother died. I've always felt a sense of love deep within. A love I thought was from my adopted mother. Now I wonder if it's Judith's love that has been with me all these years. I guess no matter where this feeling of love comes from, it adds to the pool of love from within which feeds, nurtures and nourishes us. I have such fond memories of staying with Judith and Kevin during Christmas holidays, all of us kids sitting in a circle around Kevin each night as he read the Faraway Tree, a book I read to my girls many times.

Continuing on we visit Nikki. Her home is a ship built in the 1800's to cart sugar. Entering the front door we walk straight into the enormous awe-inspiring timber hull, the cool air carrying an old musty scent. Big piles of sugar along the far side. Seamen with long hair and beards shovelling the sweet shiny crystals into hessian sacks ... well that's what I see in my mind's eye.

"This is incredible Nik. Incredible!"

"Yep, welcome to my home," she replies with a big hug and a smile as we both marvel at our surrounds and revel in each other's company.

We meet up with Corey and crew in their big van, relishing shared meals inside their spacious luxury. With a few more days of enjoyable travelling but disappointing surf we are all glad to head south, where we are met with a dreamy fantasy of corduroy lines, calmly and consistently rolling along the point breaks. Hallelujah! We spend the week relaxing in this surf haven. We meet up with Bill, who has been in the line-up surfing ten foot waves along the headlands all week with his friends, while we were in the traffic line-up!

Exploring some of the back beaches, we travel along narrow dirt roads hugging the steep hills with sheer drops to the side. It seems Corey's fancy plush van is taking up both sides of the road, much to Yasmin's dismay, leaving no space for oncoming cars. Now it's our turn to have a good laugh as our little van sneaks comfortably around the corners.

In the last days of our trip *another* cyclone hits New Zealand. Our plans to surf the East coast are stifled when Cyclone Cook has the whole area under alert with slips, flooding and many roads closed. Instead, we have an extra day in Auckland to poke around in search of my birth father. Except that I forgot it's Good Friday and all offices and registries are closed. Instead the girls and I visit my uncle, a man who is no doubt most like my grandfather, the deacon of the church who sent me away. A feeling of dread sweeps across me. I'm expecting an ultra-conservative god-fearing man to be looking down on me as Jemma, Lily and I walk towards his old house. We stop in surprise when a man suddenly appears at the window, peering down from the second storey.

"Come round the back," he smiles, signalling to the pathway down the side.

I almost gasp when I see him, his wispy grey hair melding into enormous side burns.

I whisper, "He looks like …"

"Count Olaf! A Series of Unfortunate Events," Lily choruses.

"Yes!" we all agree. "It's spooky."

Large sleepers dangle from both ears. How very odd, he has the exact same piercings Jemma and Lily have, which I have complained about numerous times. His knitted vest looks like it was created years ago. This is *not* what I was expecting!

Almost immediately I feel love for this caring light-hearted man. I am burning with curiosity to know more about him but dare not ask too much in the short time we have. Is he the black sheep of the family? There must be a good few stories behind those piercings and unruly hair. He and his wife mention my mother being here when she was pregnant with me, which gives me a strange feeling to know I've been here before. A place where I experienced pain and rejection, but now I have received love and acceptance. I gratefully accept this as another gift of unexpected healing.

Di Ellis

The next day sees a calm flight and a beautiful two-hour sunset back home. It seems the universe always has a plan. What a surprise to meet such a lovely man walking in the shoes of my grandfather. A man who I so dreaded and despised. I am learning that healing happens in so many varied and unexpected ways. Sometimes, without us even realising.

25 Healing at Warp Speed

Every day the blissful relief from Lyme symptoms continues. After years of suffering agonising symptoms daily, who would have thought bicarb soda would provide almost total relief! But I need to take the bicarb daily to sustain that relief, and my intention is to be completely free of Lyme altogether. And there's still the rather troublesome problem of suspected cancer, which needs to be cleared also. In fact, it's only in those damaged areas where any Lyme symptoms reappear when I don't use the bicarb. It's well known that Lyme thrive in damaged areas of the body. As those areas in my body diminish so do the areas affected by the Lyme. I meet a man also having great success with bicarb who emphasises the benefits of using magnesium on the skin. While I have been reluctant in the past due to reports that Lyme thrive on magnesium, I also know many Lyme patients are too low in magnesium for that reason, so I give it a go. Once again another improvement in my energy levels and relaxation.

Oxygen therapy, including the use of hyperbaric chambers, keeps coming to my attention. I remember a man named Neil who I met at a conference on the Gold Coast and wish I still had his card. I keep feeling I'll be working with him in some way. With my back much better than it's been in a long time, I give the whole house a spring clean. Low and behold Neil's card appears in an unexpected place. I go to his website where I'm drawn immediately to Genome Healing. Neil's work partner Carol Roberts has developed these techniques over years, incorporating a variety of teachings and experiences from all over the world. The video testimonies look too good to be true with seemingly miraculous healings, but one man who shares his experience is a chiropractor I used to see. Someone I trust. He highly recommends this practice.

I attend the basic and advanced courses. After just one day I know this form of healing is like nothing I've ever experienced before. Genome Healing I discover is a direct simple way to access and transform our deepest feelings at a cellular level. It does so in a way that is profound. Part of the therapy is listening to the feminine and masculine energy of every cell, organ or system of the body. We also release traumas, including ancestral trauma, genetic memory and past events. Then the incredibly powerful, yet simple process of transformation back to the creator's perfect blueprint. Wow!

I notice a lot of people are having big physical and emotional healings. Having already done such a huge amount of work on the emotional traumas in my life I'm not really having any big deep moments of awakening. It just feels normal like putting on a favourite old glove. The process fits perfectly. Doing this work in the group and pairs, I'm happy my input and understanding of the human psyche is very much appreciated. When listening to the feminine and masculine energy of my brain and heart the emotions which surface are not surprising.

I am though very surprised when we get to the gallbladder. I'm expecting something to do with anger, but to my surprise an emotion that I've never noticed before appears. I have a sudden feeling of being lost. No grief. No fear. Just lost and not knowing where I am. With my eyes closed I stay with the feeling, observing and watching it. It feels like it's around the time after my adopted mother died. I have dealt with so much grief and fear around that, but this is different. It's about my place and orientation in the world. Hmm, very curious. Once connecting with the depths of these emotions we do the transformational process back to the creator's perfect blueprint, and as usual a complete feeling of wholeness and oneness descends.

It's toward the end of the advanced course that my really big 'aha' moments occur. One process I've been waiting for is the transformation of viruses and bacteria. I'm invited out the front where I'm directed through the seemingly bizarre process of talking with the consciousness of the Lyme bacteria. I feel the writhing spitting anger of this illness in my body. My head is heating up, burning almost. Carol invites the bacteria to participate in the transformation process but it couldn't care less about the effect it's having in my body and is very comfortable just where it is. With Carol's gentle persuasion the bacteria agree and we go through the steps. I have a very clear vision of the Lyme transforming into white blood cells and I feel very positive about the process. To my surprise for the next two days I feel no symptoms at all, for the first time in over seven years. Some symptoms do return, but I know the process has been profound.

With a partner we do another process to eliminate any disease or illness. Sitting towards each other I'm receiving the healing and my partner is facilitating. Neither of us have ever done this before. With my eyes closed I visualise the process she is talking me through. I begin feeling sensations in my body that I'm not having any control over. What's going on, I wonder. I suddenly realise, inside my body, I can feel the process she is talking me through. My partner isn't touching me. She's just moving her hand a foot or two in front of my body. This is so bizarre. I'm used to being in control of what I think and feel, but this is happening without me trying. I happily sit back and enjoy the process. To my sheer amazement at the exact moment my partner says she's removing the first renegade cell from where the problem began, I feel a sharp sensation in the area of the scar on my back, and in the corresponding reflexology point in my foot. I am truly amazed.

It just so happens that during this week of training I'm due for my six-monthly thermal imaging check-up and it's only just down the road. I'm not expecting miraculous findings but with being on the bicarb over the past six months I've felt huge improvements, and with all this healing I've been doing I'm hopeful for good results. Sure enough I'm very happy to find some areas are unchanged, some have improved and some have completely resolved. Brilliant!

Back at training I have asked a number of questions, again my birth mother coming to my attention. I feel resentment for not being given the full name of my father and therefore being unable to meet him, especially as he moves into his later years. Seeing this as a good demonstration opportunity for the class Carol invites me to the front again. She tells me to close my eyes and asks me a number of questions. I share the overall story that my grandmother wanted to keep me, but grandfather wouldn't allow it and the events that followed. Carol is gently questioning, allowing me to become in touch with all of my feelings around this topic. I mention a few traumatic events, my beliefs and feelings. I feel quite relaxed about it all. Just the same, we do a trauma release for all of the events that occurred during that time. No deep grief, but the process enables a much lighter feeling. I wonder if maybe I have dealt with everything to its core as we are not really finding much to enable a shift. With one question this changes dramatically. Carol asks me if I would like to become my mother. With Carol's direction I try to say, "I am my mother", but I can't even finish this short statement due to the grief that instantaneously overwhelms me, crippling me forward on the seat. "I always wanted to keep her," I hear myself weeping.

Once again I have become deeply aware of my mother's feelings, held within me since before I was born. I feel tissues placed gently into my hand, which I gratefully use to catch my river of tears. My whole abdomen is clenched tight, curling me up, pulling me to the depths of my being, to the source of this profound deep grief overflowing from within. Eventually the grief subsides. Carol takes us both, my mother and I in spirit, through the transformer process. This enables a very deep sense of peace and contentment as I breath a huge sigh of relief.

The next day I take up Carol's offer of help during the lunchbreak, to work through my feelings around my birth father. I've come to the conclusion I probably won't meet him and have found peace with that. More than anything I want to resolve the patterns that keep me from meeting a man and having a relationship. My soul mate. Someone to walk beside me in life. I have no doubt I'm restricted by something to do with my father, I just don't know exactly what it is or how to overcome it.

Carol talks with me, implementing a few processes. We explore my feelings within. During the transformation process an image comes to my mind. My father and I and our whole community become a tribal community. Instead of us being clouded in shame we are embraced and it's okay for my father to love me. Just like I did with my mother, I speak as my father. Carol asks me some questions and I hear my father's voice through mine, telling me how sorry he is that he was never able to be there for me. This whole process no matter how real or not, is deeply profound and creates a very real shift within me, enabling a sense of connection with my father and a feeling of being loved by him. While I experienced a deep sense of soul love from my father during past breathwork sessions, I now feel a shift on a physical cellular level in my body.

What's quite incredible and very real is that one week later I meet an Islander, a tribal man who I have an immediate and mutual connection with. I am welcomed into his family and the whole vision in my healing is now a reality in front of my eyes. He rings me every night asking when I'm going to come and visit and spend time with him, his brothers, sisters and cousins and so on. I want so much to do so but I cannot, for I discover he is married. His wife has been away for a long time. He is lonely and doesn't want to see me being lonely either. This is so strange. What's going on? These are exactly the feelings and circumstances surrounding my father.

I now see a man who openly and deeply cares about all of his friends and family members, making sure each person is looked after. My mind and body are in turmoil. I feel like I'm being pulled in two. I crave so deeply to be with this man, but I know I can't. I don't know what has happened, but I know this is something very powerful. Something beyond my understanding or comprehension. As much as my mind wants to judge and say this is wrong, this man has given me something very special, deep and primal. I don't really understand what it is or how this has happened, but I know without doubt I need to accept and appreciate it, whatever it is. In doing so, something inside me awakens. For the first time in my life

I feel like I have accepted the part of me that is a part of my father, a creative and primal lifeforce energy. My goddess within, a deeply feminine and passionate side to myself, has arisen. The fire within her burning brightly, possibly for the first time in this lifetime.

A few weeks later I come down with a bit of a cough and the right-hand side of my throat where my tonsil used to be is sore. Suddenly I remember that I have some missing parts! I forgot that. One of the techniques of Genome Healing is to bring back the consciousness of any missing organs or body parts. With curiosity I do the process of bringing my missing tonsils back. I acknowledge and listen to the left and right tonsils. The left is quite happy and content. The right ... that's another story.

"There is NO WAY I'm coming back into that body and why the hell do you even want to stay there?" I hear a voice in my head saying. It takes a lot to convince the 'tonsil' to agree to participate in the transformation process, but finally it does. I do a trauma release to alleviate any shock from the operation when the tonsil was removed. This provides a surprising feeling of relief in my body. As soon as the whole process is finished I feel a gentle deep sensation in my right side, almost a feeling of fullness and being more present in my body. I feel a very strong and blissful movement of energy in my body. How very strange.

Since the Genome Healing processes so many things have suddenly shifted in my life. So much moving forward, releasing this feeling of being suppressed and held back, which has stifled me for so many years. I feel like my physical, emotional and spiritual healing has been accelerated to warp speed. I would hope for total spontaneous healing, which I know is possible after hearing so many experiences such as those of Anita Moorjani, but for some reason I seem to need the physical remedies. I wonder if it may be a reminder that I need to be grounded in this physical body. Something that has been very difficult for me. As often happens once I have worked on the emotional or spiritual level, another helpful remedy comes to my awareness. But when I say physical remedies the one I am about to experience is actually energy medicine in a physical form.

I meet a lovely lady named Elizabeth at the Genome course and I book in for a bio-resonance session with her. Once again this is similar to the treatment with my German doctor many years ago, and Dr Clark's work, but with updates in technology it's quite incredible what can now be done. I hold two copper rods with wires going into a small metal box attached to a computer which has a database of the frequencies of thousands of substances. Elizabeth programs a scan and within minutes the machine has monitored the levels of hundreds of substances in my body. She then checks for many things including detoxing, bacteria, viruses, parasites, mould and even unresolved emotional traumas. There are some things slightly out of balance, but a short rebalancing with the machine and the next results show my body has responded well.

When Elizabeth tells me that I've really done a lot of work, I'm surprised that the machine can detect that. Nothing is showing up as a major problem. No emotional traumas showing up, some mould but quite low levels compared to most people I'm assured. Though Lyme is not showing up, the machine detects that my body is responding well to the frequencies to treat Lyme. There are signs of past infections with some very strange viruses such as parvo, a dog virus, and myxo, a rabbit virus. No doubt from the tick bites. Immediately the MMS1/CD and MMS2 comes to my mind. I have no doubt these remedies, so highly recommended by Jim Humble and Kerri Rivera, with their strong oxidizing mechanisms, have killed many of the pathogens in my body and I'm relieved what a great job they seem to have done. Once all the scans are complete Elizabeth puts a small homeopathic bottle on a metal pad. Through this pad all of the frequencies that my body responded well to for further balancing are sent into the bottle from which I take a dose twice a day until my next appointment. The next day after waking I feel quite a shift. I'm not sure what it is, but something is different. Once again another step forward.

In the past when I've had urinary tract infections it often goes to the bladder and kidneys causing me extreme illness and agony. With a recurrent bout of UTI's many of my natural remedies including MMS1 don't seem to be doing the trick, which surprises and disappoints me. I really don't want to take antibiotics after all the good work I've done to balance. Instead I have a go at the full dose of MMS2 as recommended by Jim Humble. The results are almost immediate giving me huge relief. Within ten to fifteen minutes I also feel it working in the areas of concern in my back. This encourages me to stay on high doses since it's Jim's most recommended protocol for cancer and also good against Lyme. Once again, I feel significant improvements with a sensation of breaking down and letting go in the abnormal areas that showed up in thermal imaging. As usual it's in these areas that the only remaining Lyme symptoms seem to appear with muscle cramping and tingling which stops after taking the MMS2. In fact, it's this occasional cramping and tingling which keeps alerting me to the fact that these areas of damage still need to be addressed which I have to admit is somewhat a positive thing.

I often receive calls from people asking me what I've done to treat Lyme. In fact I can be on the computer from the moment I wake up to the moment I go to sleep answering questions from people with cancer, Lyme and all of the diseases which Lyme mimics. I have a call from a lovely guy who's really struggling with Lyme. We share our experiences and he tells me he's just received some of Dr Klinghardt's herbal cocktail. Hmm, with all of the remedies I've tried I haven't used the latest treatment recommended by the world's leading expert on Lyme disease. That I need to try.

I look up Dr Klinghardt's website, find his recommended retailer and order the Lyme cocktail. The old batman cartoon's 'BAM' comes to my mind as I feel the liposomal herbal mixture penetrating deep into my cells. I feel it working deeply in the damaged areas that showed up in the imaging like a tingling crampy feeling, but at the same time an easing of the tightness down my right side. I wake up the next morning with my spine and the soles of my feet tingling and both breasts swollen. Hmm, no breast enhancement required! I have no doubt the bacteria, either any residual bacteria that leached out from the tooth abscess, or the Lyme bacteria in these areas are being killed off. Very interesting!

Another of the many treatments that seems to be falling from the sky during this period of accelerated healing since the Genome Healing is redox signalling molecules, either in a liquid form taken internally, or a gel for the skin. I heard about it recently from a mother I interviewed. Her son was vaccine injured when he was young and subsequently descended into autism. Now an unmanageable teenage boy, he'd been placed in a care home but after six weeks of being on the redox molecules he improved so much she was able to bring him home.

I'm a little wary of the product. It seems too good to be true. I search up the science explaining how this stuff works. I listen to patients and Dr Samuelson, an atomic medical physicist who has worked to stabilise it into a usable product. Dr Samuelson is saying this could be the biggest breakthrough since penicillin. Listening to how it's supposed to work I understand how this could be so. But is it really that good?

Many diseases and illnesses have been linked to mitochondria dysfunction. Dr Samuelson explains that redox signalling molecules are a number of compounds produced by the mitochondria and act as either cellular messengers or cellular activators. They play a vital role in almost every function of our body, including repairing of cells, regenerating and replenishing, energy production, detoxification, activation of the immune system and giving our cells the messages to kill pathogens and protect against parasites, viruses and bacteria. Cell aging is also reversed. Dr Samuelson explains it is very important for optimal health to have a balance between oxidants and antioxidants, which both play a vital role in these processes. What he says about ROS, the reactive oxygen species, particularly fascinates me because it sounds as though it ties in with the oxidation mechanisms of MMS1 and MMS2. Dr Samuelson has worked to identically replicate and stabilize redox signalling molecules in a safe biocompatible salt water solution.

"When there is damage and imbalance, how do we flip the genetic switches that help the cells to rebalance?" Dr Samuelson asks. "When functioning well, the redox signalling molecules are supposed to do this." I think of all the times I've heard doctors talk about the connection between mitochondrial dysfunction, chronic fatigue, cancer and nearly all diseases and illnesses. I research the role of the mitochondria and discover these tiny inclusions in our cells, the powerhouses of our cells, are the source of ninety percent of our body's energy. They break down waste products, are vital for DNA and RNA production, and cell growth and death. If cells don't die when they should and begin to grow uncontrollably, this is how tumours begin. Defective mitochondria replicate their own damaged DNA continually perpetuating the problem. Although my health is improving very fast I cannot go without trying this one!

The redox gel is the first to arrive in the mail. I think of the GcMAF and how fast it activates the immune system, sometimes too fast. I haven't heard any warnings about the redox, but I'm still a little wary so I apply only a small pea-sized amount of the gel to my leg. To my astonishment within less than half an hour I feel a buzzing sensation in many of the cells throughout my body. This is a good buzzing sensation, unlike the Lyme symptoms. Wow! Something is really happening. Again I feel it working deep into the damaged areas. Later in the week the redox liquid arrives, so I begin taking that each day also. As usual I push the boundaries of the dosage and within a few days I'm using quite high amounts of the gel and liquid. Over the next day or so I feel different. Very different. I have sensations in my body. Very subtle and hard to describe. Feelings of my body working well in ways it has not done in many, many years.

Within minutes of rubbing the gel down my spine I feel it working deep into the area behind the scar on my back, a sensation continuing down into the area around my liver with a strange tightening through my right side. At the same time a sense of releasing and relaxing. One night I rub it all over my face. The next morning I awake my sinuses aching, a splitting headache and a weepy discharge from my eyes. Wow, I know it must be good to give a detox reaction like that. Immediately I'm reminded of when I became sick as a teenager. For years the infection in my sinuses was intense and I kept going to the doctor who gave me six weeks of antibiotics, horrendous sinus wash-outs using barbaric medieval methods, then operations, all to no avail.

I remember Dr Klinghardt mentioning something about the importance of clearing deep seated sinus infections. I ease up on the amount I use and slowly increase. It takes a month or two of treatment before the weeping from my eyes slowly eases and stops, as do the headaches, leaving my head and thinking clearer and brighter than it has been in years.

It seems each remedy I'm finding is more and more effective than the last. But this one is incredible! Wow! I suddenly realise how much it's just like what Carol talks about in the Genome Healing. A return to the creator's perfect blueprint. That's exactly what the redox is doing; providing the information, the perfect blueprint for optimum function. The physical manifestation of what Carol teaches. This is amazing. I can feel my cells and my immune system being activated, firing up, destroying and repairing as they would normally do when functioning ideally.

A new stronger GcMAF cream with biopeptides has become available. Although my milk kefir seems to be doing the trick I order the cream to give it a go. I'm not quite sure of the role of the peptides but learn that they too play a vital role in cell function. Sure enough I can feel how effective the GcMAF is with a profound boost to my immune system and strong tingling through my spine. I feel the areas of irregularity breaking down quickly, leaving them delicate and needing time to heal. I find I can only manage using the cream once or twice a week. I apply it early in the week so that by the weekend I'm feeling strong and able to be active again without overdoing it.

After a few months I hear from trusted sources about a con artist pretending to be a practitioner selling their own version of GcMAF. This reminds me how much vulnerable people can be taken advantage of and that we all need to be wary. I'm prompted to look into the issue more and along the way I'm very happy to be referred to Dr Ruggiero's research on GcMAF which led him to a product he calls Rerum, said to be more effective than GcMAF. Dr Ruggiero worked with Dr Bradstreet which immediately gives me confidence in his work. He states that while researching the healing properties of probiotic GcMAF yoghurt, he took the GcMAF out of the yoghurt and found it was still just as powerful. In the remaining ingredients he discovered the potent immune repairing combination of Chondroitin Sulphate, Oleic acid and Vitamin D which he called Rerum and has used it to treat patients with all sorts of illnesses such as Lyme, cancer, HIV and autoimmune problems. I learn Kerri Rivera has introduced this into her protocol. She believes it is better than GcMAF with clients reporting no herxheimer reactions. No doubt another treatment for me to trial in the near future.

With my collection of favourite remedies, at times I feel a little confused when to use each one. I have read reports that bicarb neutralizes MMS1/CD so I need to take them separately. The fermented drinks can't be taken at the same time as the MMS or anti-microbial herbs, but can benefit from lower levels of stomach acid when taking bicarb. I have used a pendulum before without much success, but decide to give it a go for some guidance as to which remedies to take and when. My orgonite pendant does the trick. I don't remember which way is supposed to be yes or no so holding the pendulum I state my name. The pendulum swings anti clockwise. I then state my name is George. To my surprise, almost immediately it swings back and forth. I play with this for some time until I feel very confident of the process. As much as I think it's airy fairy it seems to be giving some surprising accuracy.

I state, "Bicarb is the best for me at this time." The pendulum swings back and forth. "MMS1 is best for me now. MMS2 is best for me now." The pendulum begins moving anti-clockwise. To double check I state, "MMS2 is not best for me now." The pendulum swings back and forth but returns to an anti-clockwise movement when I again state that the MMS2 is best for me now. I continue listing all of the remedies and narrow it down to the MMS2 and the redox gel for this afternoon. Each day I check and double check what the pendulum says. While I'm in awe of its accuracy I will never rely on it 100%. Common sense and intuition still hold a strong footing. By monitoring the way I'm feeling each day and how each remedy is affecting me I create my own very happy and successful protocol, which is always subject to change.

Since being on the redox signally molecules, the redox gel and rubbing it all down my spine, I can feel it working within minutes of applying. I'm feeling a very sudden and distinct increase in the strength in my back, able to do more and more each day, with less and less symptoms. I don't really feel a lot when taking the redox liquid so I just keep to the gel. I also notice I can do much more with less crash in energy and vitality. In fact the improvement in my back is astounding. Since Lily moved away the lawns are only mown on her visits home. This has been one job I certainly was not going to attempt while my back was bad, especially due to the action needed to start the mower. With summer rains providing ideal growing conditions and my back feeling good, it's time to tackle this tick breeding environment. Very carefully holding my back straight and strong I pull the starter cord. A few pulls and nothing. I change hands. A few more pulls and the mower finally starts … Done with no problem! I feel a huge sense of accomplishment. I mow the front yard with success and can't help begin cleaning up a section of the garden, weeding, cleaning, lifting and raking.

I feel like I'm in a joy-filled dream, carrying out these simple tasks without pain in my back. I have a few small niggles and once again I know I've probably overdone things a little, so I save the rest for another day. Although there don't seem to be many ticks around, I immediately shower to be sure. I rub a large amount of the redox gel down my whole spine and the next day I'm feeling much better than expected. The next week I mow the back yard, do some more gardening and look around in sheer joy at what I've achieved. This yard with its lawns and gardens represents the physical effort I have just put in to clean them up and all of the inner strength, trust, hard work, treatments and methods of recovery I have used to be able to achieve it. I also have no fear of more ticks due to the effectiveness of the treatments I have to eliminate their toxins.

For four or five months I've been using the redox gel, continually increasing the amount. I finally reach a point, which I can only describe as critical mass within the cancerous cells. I can feel them breaking down dramatically, so much so that I almost feel like I'm falling apart, in a good way. I also notice my menstrual cycle affected and presume there is some sort of repair process going on. I realise I need to stop using the gel to allow my body to detoxify what is breaking down. To repair and strengthen. I think I will have a break for a couple of weeks and then start again. I use the pendulum and it seems to agree with me when I say to wait three weeks. I continue with the full dose of MMS2, which I have no doubt is providing continual improvement. I test and retest using the pendulum each day to see if and when my body is ready to start again. Sure enough after the three weeks is up, it begins to turn clockwise.

Now I decide to use the redox liquid again. This time I feel a dramatic change internally. I begin to realise that I preferred the gel before because I could apply it directly to my whole spine and felt it working in the damaged areas which were of greatest concern. Now I feel the liquid working deeply and within a week or so many areas are once again feeling like they are breaking down. The area going from the scar on my back all the way through my body to the front right side under my ribs near my liver, the right side of my chest at the top of my breast up into my right shoulder, both feeling as though they could tear if I exert myself too much. I take it easy, allowing this breaking down and rebuilding process to take place and I continue to feel more dramatic improvements.

In the following year my friend tells me about her naturopath who sent blood tests of several cancer patients, all with differing cancers, away to test the levels of circulating tumours cells and determine which treatment, of all possible treatments including holistic and mainstream, would be most effective for each form of cancer. She was astounded to learn the redox products came out on top of the list for every cancer. Amazing.

I find myself with the opportunity to try CBD oil, the form of medical cannabis without THC which doesn't get you stoned. I am very excited. This is something I've been hearing about for such a long time, but the product is so difficult to access even though it's supposed to be legal here in Australia. One dose and I feel like a switch has been flicked within me. It's very difficult to explain. It just feels like underlying negative feelings within my body have switched off, disabled in some manner. At the same time, in a subtle way, I can feel other pathways and processes within my body have been switched on for the first time in many years. I feel hunger pangs which I haven't felt in years. Like my digestion is working again. I don't understand what is happening or why, but I don't care. I trust the doctors who have worked with these products and have faith in all of the positive experiences I've heard. I also wonder... if the underlying cause of most diseases and illnesses is parasites, viruses and bacteria maybe the miniscule amount of THC which can be found in CBD oil is getting them stoned and they just can't function!

My continued relief is enormous. I feel so good! Lily comes to visit and the surf is pumping. A solid six to eight foot. Meeting Bill at Back Beach we all paddle out in the rip excitedly looking at each other with big grins on our faces, just as we have done so many times before. As soon as a big wave comes we turn around and paddle for it. We're all on. Jumping to our feet we just manage to manoeuvre our boards down the wave without running into each other.

"Woooo yeeeeaaah! I call, racing to catch up with Bill whilst leaving Lily caught in the whitewash.

"Hurry up," I yell to Bill, who's laughing with joy watching me skim behind him on the water.

Back in the lineup a big set wave is coming. Lily's in the perfect spot. I can't help but drop in again. Mum's always have drop in rights! As I career down I dig my hand into the face of the wave helping to pull the board around out of Lily's way. I straighten up, and go as fast as I can. I hear a little squeal of excitement behind me as she races up close behind. I stall, go to the top of the wave, and allow myself to come off the back giving her a free run.

We continue for a couple of hours, dropping in on each other, sharing waves, laughing and cheering each other on. It's almost surreal. But it *is* real. So many times I've grasped onto any little improvement telling myself I'm almost better. This frame of mind certainly did help me to get through. But now, feeling these significant improvements, at ease and comfortable every day is wonderful. I look back at all the times I wanted to give up. When I was just exhausted holding on, searching desperately for answers, trying so hard but still not getting anywhere. I'm so glad I didn't give up when everything seemed so useless and I was in so much endless agony day and night, year after year. I'm so glad I kept searching, looking for remedies, treatments and healing methods. Glad that I kept opening up to my inner self, to any learnings that may be beneficial. And I continue to do so. No matter what happens in my life I look for the learning or healing in the situation. It can be difficult if it is preceded with the release of traumatic feelings, but I now know it will almost always lead me to more experiences of deeper love in my life or within myself. And each time I have released the emotional connection to physical illness a remedy or treatment method has somehow made itself available to me.

It really is vitally important to never give up. At the same time it can be just as crucial *to* give up, let go and surrender to the path we are being led along. In fact it has been many times when I have come to the point of giving up that my hope has been resurrected. We need to recognise the very delicate balance between letting go and surrendering, and never giving up. It is when we are able to achieve both that the true power of each is enabled. When we give up our will and control, and surrender to the guidance of the divine or universal energies, while at the same time acting upon that guidance, hoping and praying for the very best outcome, this is often when the true power and miracles of the universe reveal themselves to us.

26 When Worlds Collide

An endless flow of little miracles continues in my personal and professional life. I have incorporated Genome Healing techniques into my Breathwork practice and now work as a Health Coach, supporting people through their own healing journey. I'm in awe watching how easily and effortlessly traumas are released, passions ignited and lives are transformed. I often attend the Genome courses brushing up on my own skills while assisting others in their learning and healing process.

This also enables me to visit Lily more often. At the beginning of the year she took the move to study of all things, psychology. Over the years if Lily ever told me about a problem with anyone at school I always asked her to think about what would be going on for them. It gives me great satisfaction now to see her study these concepts and different ways of thinking.

I thought I'd be devastated when Lily moved out, but to my surprise it was a huge relief. There isn't a large variety of different things for teenagers to do in our small home town and I could see her looking for more excitement. So that left just me. No kids. No partner. No pets. After a lifetime of nurturing and nourishing others here I am on my lonesome. Any time in the past I'd have thought it would be the worst nightmare, but wow! It's the first time in my life I don't have to worry about anyone or do anything for anyone else. Time to simply nurture, nourish and spoil myself, and I'm loving it!

For six months or so this time to myself has been wonderful. I must say though it's barely longer than two weeks before Lily is back home or I'm up visiting her, and this time it's our birthday. Jemma has recently made the move north also. The three of us sit chatting amongst the bags, clothes, dishes and mess sprawled around this teenage room, just like we've done so many hundreds of times in the past. I'm secretly thriving, loving every moment. Nikki arrives from New Zealand and we catch up with old friends Kim and Leanne. I am thrilled! It's my birthday and I get to hang out with my close friends and both of my girls.

Lily has big plans for the evening with a dress up theme so I've pulled out an old opera singer's dress.

"Happy birthday," I hear the bouncer at the door say to Lily as he checks her ID.

"Oh, happy birthday," he repeats to me as he scans my ID.

Quantum Health

We sip our drinks and I look around at all these gorgeous faces. I can't believe I'm doing this. My liver is certainly doing well. I no longer have any problem handling a little alcohol. The girls take us to several night clubs, each providing a new variety of free birthday drinks. A part of me just can't believe this is happening. But a touch of that reckless free spirit that shut down years ago has once again awoken and is thriving on this experience, simply because I can.

By midnight Nikki and I say goodbye to Jemma and Lily at the nightclub and head to an Irish bar where we hit the dancefloor, our bodies spontaneously electric, moving freely to the rhythm as they always did. We look at each other smiling and laughing with joy. It's just like the past twenty-five years never happened.

I have a few hours sleep before I'm up and off to the Genome basic course to accompany an old friend Callum who lived through some extremely traumatic events when he was young. He told me about the dark feelings he has. He's never been able to shake them and knew they would be there always. After one session of Genome Healing, with a touch of breathwork and PSYCH-K™, he was wide eyed and very surprised to realise all those bad feelings just weren't there anymore; that he felt fantastic and really light.

I suggested he attends the basic Genome Healing course where the whole class is now witnessing the power of these techniques and miracles of healing. My own miracle of healing continues to astound me. Out all Friday night, then a big weekend of healing and interaction with beautiful like-minded souls. It seems a little contradictory, to say the least, but I have given up judging, thinking what is good or not, what should or should not be. This mixture of events has provided the most amazingly joyful birthday weekend. I'm a little tired naturally, but I'm powering on and feeling good.

While I still love and crave my private quiet times in the beautiful little coastal town I call home, I'm loving my time spent away. I'm thriving on being around all the different people, cultures, the sounds and smells of city life that tantalise my senses. Lily has now been offered a contract with a modelling agency on the Gold Coast which, by coincidence, is in partnership with the first agency I worked with in Brisbane. It was when I was her age that I had to turn down a contract because of my health. Due to university and other commitments, Lily takes this offer no further and in some way moves on from a place where I left off. Jemma puts her resume in to a few places. She walks into a bar and is given a job almost immediately. It just so happens to be the place where I met her father.

Also by coincidence my girls are living in the same area where I lived, following in the footsteps of their mother and grandmother. The energetic and spiritual ties are calling. Another full circle is complete.
It's well documented that if we have a trauma during important developmental stages in our lives, that part of us stops developing. I'm discovering that when we allow those traumas to unlock naturally, when they are ready to do so, the vibrant energetic, enthusiastic part of us that shut down at that age is also unlocked. Now while revisiting my old stomping grounds I feel like I'm returning to collect energetic parts of myself that were left behind or shut down.
Though it has dawned on me how old I've suddenly become and how much living I feel I've missed due to ill-health, I seriously feel like a teenager again. A lot of the love and vibrancy that has been supressed for so many years is just bursting from within me. The crazy fun things the universe is throwing back at me in return is hilarious. I never thought this would be happening at nearly fifty! So much so that I really need to remind myself that I'm not eighteen, and while I enjoy every moment I'd better behave myself a little! I have no idea where this ride is taking me, but I sure am enjoying it!
How wonderfully idealistic it would be to end this book with a love story. Well guess what?! I just knew it ... for years. I *knew* I would meet my soul mate in a dreamy natural setting. Not out looking for Mr Right after a few drinks in a pub or a club as I did my younger years when my abilities to discern were clouded and off kilter. I knew it would most likely be at the beach, surely in the surf, especially with all of our travels over the years surfing from Noosa to Sydney and so many places in between. That is what I thought, but how wrong I was. All these years of surf adventures and not one romantic gesture. Well maybe a look and a smile but certainly nothing of substance, nothing to hold on to. I know I wasn't ready for a relationship then but I have been for a while now.
The only problem is I am fed up. Fed up with hoping, wondering, wishing and waiting. Meeting someone and fantasising that this is going to be the love of my life for it all to dissolve and vanish into thin air before it even materialised. Since the Genome Healing it seems men have been falling from the sky with random phone calls and introductions, and of course with the bad influence of my own daughters. But no more hoping or waiting for Mr Right. I am done with it. As I point out to Nikki, one of my closest confidantes, no more emotional attachment. And for the first time in my life I really mean it. I realise I have been judging people who may just be extremely lonely and desperate for human connection. For

the first time I feel truly free to meet and enjoy the company of different men, getting to know different souls, exploring their likes and dislikes and what makes them happy in their day to day life. I feel a freedom, a detachment and independence that I've never felt before, and I really like it.

I'm invited to a movie and drinks at a wine bar with a couple of the girls. We have a lovely night and make our way to the local pub for a dance. Soon a tall, dark and handsome man has his hand in mine, twirling me around the dance floor. Time seems to disappear. I have no idea how long we've been dancing for. I feel myself spinning and twirling freely with the guidance of this charismatic stranger, his hand holding mine our deep gazing eye contact unbreaking. We talk a little and he seems really nice. "Are you married?" I ask. I can't be bothered beating around the bush with that issue.

"No!" he replies in surprise.

A couple of drinks and feeling a little haphazard I'm soon flirtatious with another suitor. Nonetheless Tall Dark and Handsome takes my number before we go our separate ways. With only just enough time to arrive home my phone rings.

"Craig here. Just checking I've got the right number," he says.

Although I cringe a little when I think of my behaviour on our first meeting, I'm happy to say that our first date is cocooned in romance. On arrival I feel awkward but I try to relax as we enjoy our meal at a beautiful French restaurant. Very quickly our conversation becomes deep and meaningful and I'm fearful of exposing my life's dramas. My attempt to lighten our discussion doesn't dampen his interest as many synchronicities in our lives are revealed. He asks where I'm from and about my family. My mind searches quickly for the simplest answer.

I mention my adoption but leave out the death of my adopted mother and quickly turn the spotlight onto him. He shares about his family and then to my surprise mentions that his mother adopted out a girl. Not only was it near to the time my mother was pregnant with me, but our mothers lived in the same city. I wonder how it is possible that I meet this lovely man in my little home town and both of our mothers grew up and adopted out a girl in the same city in another country. My whole life's story and the underlying theme of what has shaped my whole life flashes through my mind. We look at each other speechless. This moment surreal. We are both intrigued as more synchronicities reveal themselves. Following a delicious meal we walk along the beach. The moon shines brightly on the water, the headland and cliffs nearby illuminated by her gentle rays. Our arms brush and I feel his warm hand take mine. The sand soft and cool under our feet. Nearing the rocks we turn to go back. His arm reaches around my waist pulling me close. His tall strong frame holding me. His warm soft lips caressing mine.

Over the coming months I get to know this lovely man. He is the perfect mix of sensitive and gentle, yet strong and masculine. While I have felt at home with him from the moment we met, my every insecurity and fear is challenged. And eight years younger? I didn't order this! I asked for someone a few years older, maybe a little chubbier, hairier, balder or something! That would have been fine. And tall. He is so tall! I'm close to six foot and I have to look up. Yes I wanted tall but, oh my, he is gorgeous. Perfect in fact. Well, perfect to me at least. How am I going to deal with this? How will I possibly handle all of these insecurities which are flooding any sensible thought I may pretend to have? I feel the angst and tension in my body but remind myself to let go of it. To let go of those fears. To allow love and only love to fill my life. For the first time in my life I'm able to stand strong in myself, observing but letting go of the mixed emotions and energies bouncing around like a pinball inside me.

Time goes on and the more I feel for this man, the more I fear this man. When I am with him I feel so calm and at ease in our connection. But when we're apart I question if what I am feeling is real? Will it last? I feel the immense fear deeply within every cell of my body. The intensity of these fears rise to a point where I feel like I just won't be able to function. I know now to completely surrender. To allow these feelings. That is all I can do. The feelings become so intense I find myself going into a place of shock. The fear turning into a feeling of numbness, the only thing enabling me to function and get on with my days. I can now see clearly that every bit of tension I have ever held in my body is the fear of love, which is in fact the fear of losing love. I purposely don't voice my fears and doubts. I don't want to give them any respect, any energy. I only voice and share kindness, caring and love, and that is all that I receive in return. Craig's mum Jen comes to visit. He is often playing scrabble with her online so on my arrival I present a deluxe scrabble board for us all to play. I don't know if it was me or the scrabble board but it's love at first sight! The connection and bond I form with Jen is immediate and deep, both of us feeling as though we have known each other always. I find myself being pampered, nurtured, cared for and loved in ways that feel so natural and comfortable. It all seems so incredible, almost confusing, but I cherish every moment. My feelings of being in the womb flash through my mind. The huge part of me that shut down when my mother lost her lover and I lost my mother. Now I have gained both. As our parallel lives join linking perfectly together I feel like I am the missing piece of a jigsaw puzzle which has been placed nicely into position, just where it belongs, making the picture come together, whole and alive.

With these incredible feelings of deep unconditional love, the climax of sheer and utter panic sets in. What if in six months, or a year or two he is no longer interested. How can I possibly open my heart fully to this incredible love to risk losing it again? I couldn't bear going back to my life without him *and* his mother. My chest feels literally like it's being ripped apart. I can feel all the areas in my back, those abnormal, damaged areas near my heart that have been locked in fear probably all my life. I imagine the worst possible scenario and tell him that maybe I should leave and allow him to find someone more suitable. He looks at me with shock and disappointment and I quickly try to explain that it's not what I want but what I fear. Everything becomes confusion. For a few days I feel like I'm losing him. I realise I've done exactly what I always did. Running away and screwing everything up in this crazy panic.

Thankfully I'm able to pull myself together and find my deepest courage to surrender to wherever this life and love is taking me. I explain that despite my cool, calm and collected exterior, a part of me within has been severely damaged. Broken. I acknowledge that part of myself, recognising the most tender deep love within. I embrace it. I nurture it. I breathe. And then I breathe again. I take this opportunity to share this inner sacred part of myself with him. I make sure not to say what I don't want. I express only what I do want. Our relationship is taken to an even deeper level of surreal love.

Over the coming months I talk with Jen often thanking her for raising such a beautiful son and welcoming me so warmly into her life. She openly expresses her love for me and her profound gratitude that I have come into their lives. I feel nothing but loved, appreciated and cherished. I feel my whole body, every cell, tingling with immense love. I bask in these glorious sensations, in awe of this new reality I am living.

I have shared my experience of Lyme with Craig and his mum, but I'm so scared of sharing the seriousness of my full health story. How bad my back and the cancer scare has been. How much of a failure I have felt so many times in my life, my ill-health always holding me back to the point that I give up on achieving anything. I'm terrified I will be rejected. In a strange way, I'm also scared the love and acceptance I might receive will melt my heart so much that I will collapse into nothing but a teary mess on the floor. I find the courage to share what I have kept secret for many months emphasising they must *not* worry about me. That I am so well now. To my enormous relief, again I feel nothing but love and acceptance. As the weeks turn into months and a year passes I realise that every day without the love in my life that I desired, was worth every moment of the love that I now share with this caring kind and thoughtful man ... and his mother! Every day I am bathed in love, giving and receiving with bliss. It seems so strange to me, but also very plausible that maybe, just maybe Jen is my spiritual mother. Maybe she always was. I was recently told about twin flames. This connection seemed too incredible to be true, but to my amazement and delight I'm now experiencing it for myself. An endless string of seemingly impossible coincidences which continue to unfold in the most dreamlike manner. Even more than everything I have already experienced. Events and circumstances. Family names and illnesses. Ages and star signs. All these years I have swum against the tide. All I needed to do was let go and flow with it, for the universe has a plan. A divine and wonderful plan.

Keen to share her latest health improvement remedy, Diane Sommer calls me and suggests I try a herbal tablet which activates the NRF2 pathways in our body. I don't really know what she's talking about and feel I have tried all the herbs listed in the tablet and decline the offer. Over the following months she is constantly sharing how great she feels and talks about all these other people who are having great results. I tell her I'm happy to do an interview on the radio with her and her friends but decline the offer to come along to an information day they are holding. I feel they are a bit too perky and excitable about it all for my liking. Of course, I don't tell Di that. She sends me a bottle in appreciation for doing the interview and checks three weeks later how I'm feeling. I confess I haven't taken it and with frustration I figure I'd better at least give it a go, so I can tell her I have.

Within hours, that very same day, I feel energised. The next day, and the next, my energy levels increase. I go surfing and don't experience a crash in energy over the following days. I surf more and more. Still, I'm fine. I push myself until I start to crash. I remember Di saying to take two tablets instead of one if I have a detox reaction or feel low in energy. I do so and feel myself pick up again. No major crash? I find my body and the remaining areas of abnormality in my back can't keep up with the energy I have. I slow down and give my body a break but wonder how on earth this is happening. I ring Di and tell her how good I'm feeling.

'I know, this is what I've been telling you!' she emphasises.

I apologise profusely, explaining I never thought a simple herbal tablet could have such an incredible effect. I flood her with questions wanting links to information, studies, testimonies and anything that will explain why, for the first time in thirty years, I'm not having chronic fatigue crashes in energy after exercising. Yes, I've had a lot more energy since all the healing I've done, but nothing, I mean nothing has stopped me having these nasty crashes in vitality after exercise. I meet with Di and many of her friends, some who I have also known for a couple of years. They love NRF2 and report amazing recoveries from many conditions such as back pain, arthritis, depression, fatigue, lung disorders, eczema, learning disorders and much more. I am amazed.

I research and read many PubMed studies on oxidation and Nrf2. I listen to video after video, doctor after doctor, testimony after testimony. The Truth About Cancer report the effectiveness of NRF2, and the Michael J. Fox Foundation has a study looking into its effect on Parkinson's. It seems the new buzz word in health circles is NRF2! I learn that biochemist Dr Joe McCord was the first doctor to discover oxidative stress in the body and its connection to nearly all diseases, illness and injury. He worked with a team of doctors to find something that would activate our body's own antioxidants. After testing thousands of herbs they found a combination of turmeric, milk thistle, green tea, bacoba and ashwaganda does exactly that by activating the release of the NRF2 protein in our cells. Dr McCord says the NRF2 protein is then free to enter the nucleus of every cell where the DNA resides. This DNA has the master blueprint for that cell and the plans for everything the cell needs to make. When NRF2 goes into the nucleus it has access to 25,000 genes that are in the nucleus of every cell of our body. About four or five hundred of those genes have receptors where NRF2 can bind and act.

"You can think of it as a key and a lock," says Dr McCord. "The NRF2 finds the four hundred or so genes that it can modify. It binds to them. It turns on that gene. The end result is all of those genes upregulate the thing that they encode; the blueprint for the product that the cell makes."

'The blueprint for the product that the cell makes'! Again, I am reminded of Carol's Genome Healing training, returning to the creator's perfect blueprint! Incredible.

Dr McCord says he spends hours and hours every day going through what these genes are and what they do. He says that his work was developed primarily to affect three gene products, the antioxidants called glutathione, superoxide dismutase and catalase, which it did. In the last five years they now realise NRF2 does a lot more than that.

"The overall predominant theme," he says, "is the genes that help our cells survive are upregulated and the genes that are doing the damage and causing problems are being decreased."

Cardiologist Dr Benedict Maniscalco says, "When we have too many oxidants, also called free radicals, when that free radical is not neutralized it attaches any place it wants to, including the cell membrane or mitochondria. When this happens it injures a cell and the body responds by creating more pro-inflammatory molecules which always end up in a scar. Scars replace cells, too many cells replaced, replace organs. That's disease. That's the beginning of all disease. When the specific combination of these five herbs is given and the NRF2 protein is activated we start making these life-saving antioxidants, millions of them per second. There is nothing we can take in by mouth that will do that. Nothing can replace the beauty of our own cells creating their own antioxidants. It's so powerful."

The effect of the ratio of these herbs was found to be eighteen hundred times more effective than each of the herbs on their own. Dr McCord states that one molecule of Vitamin C will remove one free radical, while one molecule of our own antioxidants will remove one million free radicals.

Dr Maniscalco also describes NRF1, a combination of Acetyl L-Carnitine, Coenzyme Q10, Alpha-lipoic acid, Grape Extract and Quercetin. All of these names are very familiar as I recall them listed on many of the supplements given to me by the molecular biologist from America. NRF1, with its combination of nutrients, and amino and fatty acids, upregulates the repair and production of the mitochondria, a part of our cells which produces all of our energy at a cellular level.

"So when you give NRF1 you make more energy and you are more efficient, the cells are more efficient, so you really need the NRF2 molecule there because with more energy and more combustion, there will be more free radicals," Dr Maniscalco explains. "So it's a beautiful biochemical cycle."

I begin taking NRF1 and feel an even greater boost in energy. Over the following weeks I'm surfing, bike riding and going for longer walks. I just can't believe it. I'm always so thrilled with each improvement in my health, but I never thought I would have that vibrant feeling of youthful, limitless energy again without the following big crash, feeling like I've been hit by a bus. Well I can't say I feel it completely yet for I still don't have the strength in my body to keep up with the energy I have. But I am experiencing those feelings of boundless energy that I remember from so many years ago in my teens that I longed would one day return. I acknowledge my tendency to push myself too hard. You'd think I would have learnt by now but my passion for living an active life and my love of being in nature is so strong. I find a nice balance between exploration of my limits and nurturing self-care. My back and neck continue to loosen and strengthen with less tingling and tightness. Although I can still feel the damaged areas especially down my right side, I don't get the tearing feelings in my back now and can lift, vacuum, mow the lawn, surf and play in ways that I couldn't for a number of years. I know very good things are happening within me.

I continue taking bicarb on waking, and NRF1 and NRF2 at breakfast. Throughout the second part of the day I take MMS2, sometimes mixing it up with MMS1 and occasionally I use essential oils, usually down my spine. My friend who has some ovarian troubles notices her period coming every two weeks, something I have been experiencing. I have no doubt the powerful healing action of the redox is detoxifying and removing damaged cells. I stop using it for a little while to let things settle down.

I see an event notice in the Lyme Disease Association of Australia's newsletter about an introduction to AmpCoil technology. The creators Aaron and Geneva Bigalow, whose family suffered the devastating effects of Lyme for many years, are planning their first international launch which happens to be in Australia. I notice my friend Sharon is one of the contacts for the Sunshine Coast event. I'm very curious as Sharon has been dedicated to supporting Lyme patients for many years but rarely suggests any particular course of action. Immediately I research this device that uses sound frequency powerfully amplified into a modified Tesla coil, which in turn creates a pulsed electromagnetic field that penetrates deeply into the body. The accompanying *Betterguide* app contains over one hundred pre-designed journeys and with the latest in bioresonance technology, a voice analysis program is used to help you choose which one will be most beneficial for you.

I attend the Bryon Bay gathering where I feel an immediate affinity with Aaron and Geneva who share the depths of the suffering and loss they experienced, a story so similar to many hundreds of thousands of people all around the world. At this gathering with so many people wanting a session I don't get a turn but after just being in the room with the coil going, I wake up the next day feeling different. Later that day I am blessed to receive a beautiful healing session with Geneva, her gentle warmth and caring strengthening the comfort I already feel in her company. We connect on a soul level and have a mutual respect for the struggles and hardship we have both endured, the dedication we share to regaining health and wellbeing for ourselves, our loved ones and all of humanity. Within minutes of the device being turned on I feel a profound effect. The suspected cancerous areas in my back, abdomen, right shoulder and neck become tight with a feeling of pressure similar to the Theraphi device. I feel a sensation of energy trying to push its way through areas of blockage particularly in my neck. My tongue, two fingers on my right hand, through my back, down my right leg and part of my right foot start twitching quite strongly. It's a very weird sensation but I know something good is happening.

The next few days I feel no need to take any of my strong remedies. Just bicarb to alkalise the body, NRF2 to remove oxidative stress and NRF1 to repair mitochondria. I have always been scared to stop taking MMS or any of the antimicrobials in case the horrific symptoms of Lyme rage their fury within me once again. But now after such a profound healing I feel confident. Very confident. I feel delicate especially in the cancerous areas and tell myself I mustn't surf this weekend. That doesn't last long though. The surf is up. Bill and his beautiful new partner Sal are already in the water. Craig is keen too.

I've missed out on living life to the full for so many years. I'm fed up with missing out. I'll just take it easy I say to myself. Three surfs later and I've had a wonderful weekend. All the abnormal areas that showed up in the thermal imaging feel like they have released, opened up and could quite easily be damaged or tear if I'm not careful. I'm exhausted but ok. This was the test. A very big test. I was wary of surfing because of the delicate areas in my muscles and spine, but also because in the past Lyme symptoms would be a lot worse after exercise and I have still taken no antimicrobials. I check in with my body. Nothing. It feels like a dream. A beautiful blissful dream. My body is at peace. I am at peace.

I've been thinking about the Sunshine Coast presentation which is five and a half hours drive north. A little voice of fear within me is terrified Lyme symptoms will return. Even if they don't I know my body needs more attention. At 11 am I decide I must go and experience this gift from God again. I drive all afternoon and just make it in time. By the end of the evening I'm the very proud owner of my own AmpCoil. I literally hold it like a baby and feel the deepest love and gratitude for Aaron, Geneva, the doctors and engineers they have worked with, and all of the pioneers before them who have enabled this miraculous technology.

Quantum Health

Two weeks later the Noosa Festival of Surfing draws us back up the highway to the Sunshine Coast. The biggest competitor based surfing competition in the world, many of the best longboard surfers gather to showcase their skills, socialise and surf together. Each year I'm disappointed with my abilities and I'm lucky if I can surf two or three times during the week. Once again I resolve to take it easy and allow whatever may be. That does not last long. The surf is up. Lines of swell roll through the ocean, peeling along the headlands as they reach the point breaks. Surfers fill the car parks, changing into their swimmers and board shorts while others make their way down the hill from their accommodation. The scraping sound of boards being waxed, excited chatting and laughter fill the air. With our boards under our arms we join the procession along the pathway wrapping through the national park. Standing on the rocks at the water's edge we wait precariously for a break in the waves. Salt water rushes around our legs, splashing up into our faces as we brace holding on. A lull in the waves provides an opportunity to jump in and we paddle quickly away from the sharp rocks out to the lineup.

My small camera in hand I sit just on the edge of the break tempting fate for the close shot as the bigger set waves nearly pull me over. I put my trust and faith in these surfers' abilities as they dodge and weave their hard and heavy nine foot plus boards around me, at times with only inches to spare. Filming every wave I'm stoked with the footage I get as they race the fast sections, ducking down into barrels, the wind and spray coming off the back of the crystal clear blue wave as it curls over the surfers. Whenever I see an opportunity I paddle for waves, Lily and I sharing as many as we can. We laugh, cheer and encourage each other. Last year Lily was very happy to be the only Aussie to get into the semi-final. No such luck this year but that doesn't dampen her spirits. We catch up with friends from all over the world. Incredible surfers who come to ride this iconic surf break in one of the most beautiful parts of the world. Walking up and down the hill to and from our accommodation carrying my board is exhausting and a challenge for my back but I manage surprisingly well. Craig, my gorgeous gentleman, always carries my board if he is with me. Each day when I feel as though I won't be able to keep going I take extra NRF2 and use the AmpCoil's uplifting programs. I am completely amazed at what I've been able to do, the strength in my body and the endurance I feel. I have surfed seven times in five days. I'm shattered by the end of the week but I just haven't stopped and lack of sleep and dehydration are most likely contributing. I feel my back and right side cursing me, not really quite ready for all this, but also thankful for such improvements. And still I have not felt the need to take any antimicrobials.

Over the following months I learn the full functions of the AmpCoil. I work my way alternating through deep cleansing programs and uplifting harmonizing settings. I feel the self-healing mechanisms within my body being activated in a breaking down and regenerating process. I allow my body the time and nurturing it needs. The areas of pain and tingling in my back and limbs have decreased dramatically. At times though, I feel a deep sensitivity and tingling through my spine and limbs, occasionally waking up with tingling and numbness. This reminds me of some of my earlier remedies as they fired up my own immune system working deep into damaged areas. Now I feel things working a lot more deeply into my spine, deep into my cells on a quantum level. This is a good thing but also a dramatic reminder of how serious my condition has been. As my body consistently strengthens I realise what an incredible healing process I am going through.

Again my thoughts return to Averil, Ian, and their music. While playing at a market they were praised by indigenous people who were taken to a profound level of deep peace. Averil often discussed the power of sound and frequency being the creator of all matter in our universe. I research quantum physics and quantum field theories, first proposed in the 1920's. The discovery that all matter, every particle is purely frequency. I read about the electron field, an electron particle being a localized vibration in this field. And there being a field for every known particle, such as the guon, muon, and quark fields; the whole universe made up of fields playing an immense subatomic symphony. I think of Bruce Lipton and his colleagues and the work they do monitoring how our consciousness can affect these fields and every cell in our body. Just fascinating!

I begin taking the redox liquid which I haven't done for a while. I notice my bowel movements become a lot more regular and normal. I think back to the dental conference I went to twenty-five years ago. A doctor said that most cancer patients don't have regular daily bowel movements of at least one to three times a day. I remember thinking I wasn't regular but dismissed it telling myself it won't apply to me. I feel the redox signalling molecules repairing my cellular function, my bowels becoming more regular and I feel my body working as it was created to do. This time my period is not affected and my monthly cycle is regular.

Week by week I continue to be able to lift more, do more, go for longer and back it up the next day. And then do more again! The strength I have gained in my back is nothing short of a miracle. Craig and I are moving to be closer with his family. As our relationship continues to deepen, I notice patterns arising that are not always beneficial. I acknowledge them and listen to what is happening within me. Craig often gives me so much support that he leaves himself depleted. I encourage him to look within. I remember the differences between individuals and the way they deal with things, particularly men and women. He reminds me that I'm at the end of my book, while he is just at the beginning.

Over the couple of years we've been together he has jumped head first, putting all his faith in me, experiencing the processes I have to offer. All the while, I've reassured him things happen when they are ready, as they are meant to. And that's exactly what has happened. I'd like to say it's all been easy and smooth sailing, but occasionally it's been far from it, triggering both of our flight or fight survival mechanisms. Powerful mind/body healing processes transform lives, but sometimes it's just the day to day addressing things with sheer commitment and dedication that is needed.

Again, I see we can have all the positive intentions in the world, but if we haven't cleared the energetic charge from negative memories or traumas in our body, they may not be effective. I use any techniques I feel necessary at the time, including an exercise shared by Dr Jo Dispenser. I visualise myself actually in a future that I desire. I feel within my cells all of the feelings that future will create. It isn't long before I feel myself living my future self once again. While at times these processes seem never ending, I continue to grow happier, healthier and free from the negative constraints of my past.

In our moving process I'm in awe as I find myself with the strength to not only scrub and clean the whole house but also to lift furniture and storage boxes day after day. And then I still have the energy and strength to go for a walk or surf. I think of how much over the years I have needed to tell myself to slow things down, to take care of myself. But I'm beginning to see that having vibrant energy and a desire to be outside in nature is actually our natural state of being. I remember at school always being that child in the class who couldn't sit still, always in trouble. I think of children now who are labelled with a condition and prescribed a drug because they can't sit still. Yes, there is no doubt many have pathogens and anxiety which cause this, but how much of their natural vitality and energy is being suppressed. Somehow as a society we are conditioning ourselves to do this.

I think of the millions of people around the world affected by Lyme disease, such a crippling illness, so many of us searching for years with very few options for complete resolution. I sigh an enormous breath of relief. Finally. I am free. I am in awe of all the wonderful simple, natural and breakthrough remedies I have discovered. The powerful mind body healing techniques. And now the AmpCoil. I know we have reached the beginning of the Quantum shift so many have been hoping and praying for.

In writing this book I hope to assist others, so many who I know are struggling each day just as I have done. I've been frustrated, seemingly held back for no reason at times, but then I have a profound learning or come across another remedy or treatment that is invaluable. I look back at the incredible events that have taken place in my life and the teachings and wisdom they have provided. I feel like my whole life has become a series of serendipitous events, mysteriously linked in so many ways. Having spent years studying the mind/body connection, researching and trialling medical and alternative treatments, and speaking with hundreds if not thousands of people around the world about their experiences, to my surprise I now find myself as somewhat of an expert in many areas.

I think of all the trials and tribulations I have experienced in my life and almost can't believe it. There is deep sadness, a very deep sadness, for so much of my life lost to ill-health. So many of my youthful years gone. But I also hold profound feelings of strength and pride. For so many years I have felt almost like I'm living two lives, my inner existence filled with emotions, feelings, memories and mystical journeys through past and present. And my outer physical world where the other is hidden, fearful of revealing itself. Writing this book has been a profound step in my healing process. Not only has it been very cathartic but I have experienced incredible healings in very unexpected ways.

Wary of sharing my story I searched for someone to support me in this process. One step led to another and I met Maggie Hamilton. She was very interested in my work. I tried to hide my naïve lack of knowledge and intense insecurities, my huge lack of self-confidence and fears of exposing my inner self to the world. But what Maggie gave me was a valuable part of my healing process. She recognised something within me that not a lot of people see, either because they just don't see it or because I keep it so well hidden. That part of me that is so delicately sensitive, yet strong with so much to share. During a three-year period of editing and updating my writings she supported that strength and wisdom within me.

After many adjustments I send in my final edit. I'm confident but very nervous. A couple of days later I open the return email from Maggie. I am floored. She is thrilled beyond expectation. Reading these words it feels like I'm in one of those movies when someone's spirit suddenly gets sucked back into their body. I feel strange. As if I could collapse. In shock almost. Once again a huge amount of tension and gripping is suddenly letting go from my body. I allow it. I feel it. I realise this gripping has been holding a very sensitive part of me, a part of my spirit, away from my body, away from this physical world for not feeling safe to be here. But now that delicate part of my self has been recognised, acknowledged and understood. Suddenly, feeling safe to be here, that delicate part of my spirit now feels it has a place in this physical world to express freely and openly. I allow the feelings of shock to release from my body while at the same time I feel the merging of my soul and my physical self.

It takes me a while to fully comprehend what has just happened. It's almost like Maggie played the role of spiritual midwife! Again this feeling of the midwife being the guide and protector allowing the natural course of events to unfold as they are meant to do. And that is how I feel about the birth of my book. Held within, as I bare my soul, are my deepest, darkest and most joyful feelings and memories, all representing those most sensitive and delicate parts of myself. With no pressure or judgement, Maggie provided gentle guidance and a warm, safe and encouraging environment enabling the full expression of my deepest inner self.

I have always felt the need to separate those two sides of myself, those deep inner feelings and experiences, and the reality of my physical world. I guess when others didn't understand what I was experiencing I felt as though it must not be real. But the more I listened to speakers such as Dr Bruce Lipton, who explains so easily how our emotions regulate our gene expression, Anita Moorjani who died at the end stage of cancer but had a full recovery soon after her near death experience, and Dr Eben Alexander who recalls his healing and incredible journey into the afterlife, the more I realise it is our inner world, our own consciousness that is just as real, if not more so than our physical existence. Ultimately, they are all created from love. I see clearly now what they are talking about, that our inner reality actually creates our physical experience. As I change my inner reality and open to the deepest love of myself and others I am seeing my outer world manifest into the most wonderful experiences.

Di Ellis

When we follow what our soul wants and loves, rather than what we think we want or what we should do, life falls into place and flows much more easily. Passions are ignited, energy is unlocked and a deeper meaning and purpose fills our life. If a hurdle comes into our path, it may well be a nudge to push us onto a different path, onto our true life's path, or into a different more suitable way of thinking. It seems the more resistance we have to travelling that path, the bigger the push we receive to redirect us. The saying 'what we resist will persist' is very accurate.

At the same time it's incredible how quickly negative feelings or circumstances can shift when we surrender to our life's path. A path which can fill us with joy almost instantly, just as it was designed to. Remember, if your negative emotions don't clear effortlessly using gentle methods to clear them, beneath those feelings lies a precious gem that is worth digging for, just waiting to be discovered. Surrender to those feelings. Follow those emotions to their depth. Treat them as your friend. Allow them to reveal the delicate love and sensitivities below, just waiting to be nurtured and treasured.

The universe will always bring the experiences we need to grow and develop, pushing us to find and unlock any areas of ourselves that have been shut down. Sometimes we can't do it to the full depth needed using a form of therapy. At times we need those real-life experiences to truly feel the experiences to their depth. Maybe, just maybe, that is what life is all about. Our lives are guided by a divine force. A love that resides within each of us, within everything in our lives. Fully and completely surrendering to and trusting this divine force which underpins all of creation is the challenge. At times if there was a problem with someone I could talk to them, dig my heels in and work hard to resolve the issue. Sometimes problems which overwhelmed me, with no resolution in sight no matter how hard I tried, I had to let go of, surrendering them to the universe, asking "Please, you just fix this for me. It's just too hard." To my surprise the negative situations or relationships I was holding onto for fear of losing them were transformed. Either that person or situation left my life or, given the opportunity to heal, came back to me filled with more love than I could have imagined.

Surrendering and trusting is like floating down a river, rather than swimming against it. The feelings in our body will take us places. Very deep places. Even to different dimensions at times. Know that every negative feeling in your body is a message. Either a warning that something is wrong and needs your attention, or guidance prompting you to go within and connect with the deeper parts of yourself. The deeper love that exists within all of us. Those two possibilities are actually one and the same, for it is when we are disconnected from our true self and the deep love within, that we are vulnerable to unhappiness or illness.

It is so fundamentally important to listen to yourself, your own intuition and divine guidance about what is most important for you at this moment. Whether it be a direction to take in your life or a method of healing to use. There are countless methods of healing, in both complementary and modern medicine, and so many wonderful forms of therapy. Some may be useful now, while others may be useful at a different time. Some methods may hinder you at present but may be very beneficial in the future.

More than anyone else, deep within, you know what is best for yourself. This principle applies to every aspect of your life including relationships and work. Parents, particularly mothers, know what is best for their children. First though you need to be connected to your intuition, your inner wisdom. By following those intuitive instincts and listening to your body you will know which path to take. If you head in a certain direction and notice yourself feeling extremely anxious or your body feels weak, listen to your body. Are you feeling fearful even though you know this is the best way to move forward? Or is your inner self, your higher wisdom, rejecting this option knowing it is not right for you? Remind yourself that despite your fear, despite what other people may think is best for you, you *do* know what is best for yourself. As Louise Hay said, listen to your 'inner ding', that light bulb that goes off within when you know something is right. Most of all, trust yourself!

Walking along the beach I look out at the ocean. I admire the powerful waves we've been riding. The dumping shore break out front and a beautiful long peeling left hand break to the south. I look up at the cliffs. The swirls of varying colours never fail to draw me in. The ice cream chocolate, coffee, toffee, and butterscotch browns blending into vanilla cream and white. The patterns created thousands of years ago being revealed by the weather, wind and waves. As I look around I no longer feel fear. Only love. No more nightmares. Only dreams. I look at my love, my tall dark and handsome, walking beside me. He teases me and smiles, his eyes looking into mine, deep into my soul. How I love this cove. How I love this life.

Part 2

Summary of My Healing Protocol

What I Wish I Knew Then

Is it possible that a few simple home remedies can save your life when you are seriously ill? Can some of the most highly advanced atomic medical research provide simple answers to reactivate and repair our immune systems and our own self-healing abilities? Can a highly sophisticated yet simple electrical device bring harmony to every cell, organ and system within our body?

Here I share a summary of the simple steps which have helped me to overcome a lifetime of chronic and serious health conditions. Chronic illness is epidemic. Every day, people are desperately searching for answers to find relief from agonizing, life-threatening symptoms.

I do not give medical advice but I happily share information which I have gathered during my healing journey. Some of these methods are commonly used, some are considered alternative or controversial, while others are ancient time-tested natural and home remedies. The methods and techniques that I mention might not be suited to some people, but I have complete faith in these remedies and methods due to the dramatic improvement they have provided for my health. I also share simple yet powerful techniques I have discovered to release the emotional connection to physical illness.

When someone is seriously ill or in agony every day, the priority is to treat the physical body. I have seen as many mainstream, natural and holistic doctors, specialists, and practitioners as I possibly could and have used thousands of dollars worth of remedies and treatments. A number of these saved my life. Some of the most simple methods were the most effective to help me regain health and provide desperately needed relief. Please note, the information below is purely for informational purposes. I trust it is helpful. I recommend you find a holistic or biomedical doctor who can assist you in your healing process.

Hidden Causes of Chronic illness

Many doctors and scientists have found pathogens to be the underlying cause of many diseases and illnesses. Dr Hulda Clark devoted her life's work to researching and removing the underlying causes of disease and illness. She correlated certain parasites, viruses, bacteria and toxins to particular diseases. Dr Clark then used simple methods to remove these from the person's body enabling a partial or full recovery. Removing pathogens is also the basis to Jim Humble's protocols (see Eliminate Pathogens).

When we remove the underlying causes of disease our body can make a dramatic recovery. However, if our immune system has been damaged or severely weakened, using methods to repair and activate our body's own self-healing mechanisms may be needed (see Activate Your Body's Own Self-Healing Mechanisms).

Biomedical imbalances, including genetic predispositions, are linked to many health conditions (see Balance Biochemistry). There can be numerous side-effects to medications and many deaths have occurred due to wrong medications.

Louise Hay supported many people to improve their health by removing negative thoughts and beliefs linked to specific diseases and illnesses.

- Biochemical imbalance
- Pathogens
- Trauma or stress (past or present)
- Negative subconscious thought patterns or beliefs
- Wrong medication

Hidden Causes of Anxiety and Depression

The previous list also applies to anxiety and depression. Dr William Walsh can look at someone's blood chemistry and determine with accuracy what mental health disorder they may have. Parasites, viruses and bacteria can get into every part of our body including our nervous system and create severe anxiety which is never ending. Biochemical imbalances and pathogens have also been linked to ADD, ADHD, learning disorders, autism and suicidal and self-harming tendencies. Dr Walsh states that some people, depending on the methylation processes in their body, can do well on anti-depressants while others can become worse or even suicidal.

There is no doubt trauma and stress create anxiety. Breakdowns can often lead to a personal or spiritual awakening of sorts (see Emotional and Soul Healing), but when anxiety and depression consistently affect everyday life it's worthwhile exploring the possibility of pathogens and biochemical imbalances, eg zinc deficiency leads to high copper which is linked to depression (see Balance Biochemistry).

As a mind/body therapist I support people to transform negative thoughts, beliefs and traumas. But if someone has persistent anxiety along with physical symptoms, particularly gut trouble, I always insist they consider pathogens as an underlying cause of their inability to process their emotions effectively or relieve the tension and anxiety in their body (see Eliminate Pathogens).

Caution and disclaimer
This is not medical advice. There is no medical advice contained in this book. Everything I share is purely for informational purposes. For professional medical advice please consult a qualified health practitioner. I have learnt about things I would rather not know, for example, greedy people and organisations that put profits way above the health and wellbeing of other people. Many of these people are happy to slander and criticize scientifically validated treatments to increase the sales of their own toxic medications. While some of the protocols I have used have been strongly criticized or ridiculed, they have saved my life and helped me to regain optimum health. Many are very inexpensive and affordable to everyone.

When I was seriously ill and dying I was sent home from hospital with anxiety medication and no further help. I was desperate. I had spent years eating a healthy diet and being very careful with anything I put into my body. When a health professional suggested I look into MMS and Jim Humble's protocol I thought it was crazy. After doing my own research I felt wary but confident to give it a try. I am so happy I did. While I discuss my experiences and what I choose to do when confronted with a health situation, I do not recommend this or any other remedy, treatment or method. Like all medications, some of the remedies and treatments I have used and talk about can be harmful if taken or used the wrong way.

KISS – Keep it Simple Sweetheart!

The most simple and effective steps to healing
Ahead I detail of all the remedies and treatments I have used, and some that I haven't but are recommended. This list is extensive and potentially very confusing. Therefore, in this **Basic Protocol** I share a few of the most simple home remedies, medical breakthroughs and methods which have provided the most relief and improvement in my health.

Aim for little or no medications or supplements
Some medications or supplements may be necessary. But, when we remove what is harming our body, replenish what is needed, and activate our body's own self-healing mechanisms, we shouldn't need to be taking countless medications and supplements. Our body is an amazing compilation of finely tuned systems capable of creating almost everything it needs for regeneration and vitality. Be open to exploring how much your body can heal itself and how strong and vibrant you can be. I know people in their eighties who have changed their diet and their blood pressure dropped to normal levels. They worked with their doctor to decrease blood pressure medication according to their health needs.

Basic Protocol ... Step by Step

This is a combination of techniques and treatments used by a number of doctors and healers. They are not my techniques. They are simple methods I have found to be most helpful for regaining optimum health and have been used by people wanting to overcome minor conditions and serious life-threatening diseases. There are many different treatments and remedies that may be more suitable for you. This is what has been the most effective for me. I highly recommend finding a biomedical doctor or naturopath to assist you in your healing.
I wish I knew about these methods when I was seriously ill and dying. Unfortunately, my condition was undiagnosed and I was sent home from hospital barely able to walk, sleep or eat and diagnosed with anxiety. I went to every doctor and natural practitioner I could. I reacted badly to almost every pharmaceutical medication and natural remedy I was given. I also reacted badly to every piece of food I put in my mouth and anything I put on my skin or breathed in. I now know my liver was congested causing these bad reactions. It was a living hell which gave me the passion to share this information with others. Due to the relief and improvement I gained, not only is this what I would do if I had my time again, these remedies are the basis of my ongoing protocol now.

Slowly and gently is the way to go
Early on my body would not have handled the detox or die off reaction from some of the remedies when pathogens are killed and the immune system is fired up. Cleansing the kidneys and liver is definitely the first step no matter what condition you have.

Quantum Health

1   Kidney and liver cleansing teas

One teaspoon of alfalfa leaf tea seeped in a mug of hot water half an hour before breakfast and dinner saved my life when I was seriously ill. My liver flushed out and my body slowly began functioning properly again. This process is very gentle and effective. A number of different herbs can be used as a tea to flush out the kidneys and liver as listed. From my experience and the recommendations of many health professionals, cleansing the kidneys and then the liver is the most important first step anyone should take when beginning treatment for any health condition. If the liver is congested it will not filter the blood effectively having a negative effect on every area of the body. As I experienced, this may not show up on blood tests. Kidney and liver cleansing teas can be bought online or in health shops (see Detox).

Dr Clark - drclark.net
Dr Sandra Cabot - liverdoctor.com
Mullum Herbals - mullumherbals.com.au

2   Bicarb soda or hydrogen water to alkalize the body

Parasites, viruses and bacteria cannot survive in an alkaline environment. Bicarb soda provided almost immediate relief of agonising Lyme disease symptoms, including continual pain and cramping in my muscles. It also minimised the symptoms of herxheimer reactions. Before I took bicarb, thermal imaging confirmed abnormalities of suspected cancer in many areas of my body including my back, spine and both breasts. Due to the enormous amount of relief I gained using the bicarb that is all I took for six months. My next results showed some areas the same, some improved and some completely resolved.

While there is a belief taking bicarb is not good due to its neutralizing effect on stomach acid, the profound relief I had outweighed the possible side effects. Simply dissolving bicarb in water and spraying on the body was incredibly effective to reduce muscular pain, tension and anxiety. Following recommendations, I took one teaspoon four times a day, forty minutes to one hour before food. Starting with a smaller amount may be required (see Alkalize Your Body).

3   Diet

A basic diet of whole fresh vegetables, some fruit, and protein is the way to go. When I cut grains out of my diet I noticed big improvements.

I have explored with many diets including vegan and vegetarian but really struggled. I have found that I do best on the paleo type of diet. Fermented food and drink provide beneficial bacteria which is crucial for gut health (see Diet/Gut Health). Drink filtered or purified water: clarencewaterfilters.com.au   mmsaustraila.com.au

4   Positive Intentions and Stress Release
When we're stressed our body is in fight or flight mode. This will create tension in the muscles restricting blood flow, and cause our cells to be in protection mode rather than repair and regenerate. Even if you don't feel it is possible, set intentions and positive affirmations about being well, such as; my body can heal and repair in every way, I am strong, healthy and well. This will create a healing effect on a cellular level and help to calm and relax your body (see Emotional Healing).

5   Kerri Rivera's CD(MMS1) protocol
Kerri has a very gentle protocol for extremely sensitive, chronically ill people. She addresses the pathogens which are often the underlying cause of most disease and illness. She also provides simple natural ways to detoxify and replenish the body. She details all the steps in her book *Healing the Symptoms Known as Autism (second edition)*.
Jim Humble also has health recovery protocols which I found very beneficial. For acute conditions or if I have been bitten by a tick I use Kerri and/or Jim's protocols (see Eliminate Pathogens).
These protocols have received a lot of criticism from people who have either not followed directions, and/or from what I believe are powerful, competing companies with a vested interest. I have spoken to hundreds of people with different conditions that have used MMS1/CD with great success at minimal expense and only minor herxheimer reactions if taken strictly to protocol. I do not recommend that you use these protocols. I am simply sharing what has been beneficial for me and no doubt saved my life.
cdautism.org   ketokerri.com   jimhumble.co

6   Repair the immune system
There is nothing more powerful and effective at healing our body than our own immune system. These steps are advised to be taken slowly. Each one of these products can fire up our immune system dramatically, potentially causing a reaction when our own immune

mechanisms attack pathogens or unhealthy cells (see Activate Your Body's Own Self-Healing Mechanisms).

NRF2
From the day I began taking NRF2 thirty years of chronic fatigue disappeared. Yes, for me this was a miracle. Dr Joe McCord found that oxidative stress and damaged mitochondria are linked to the beginning state of all disease and illness. He and his team worked to develop NRF2 which regulates gene expression; upregulating helpful genes and downregulating harmful genes. Some of these genes are involved in the production of our body's own antioxidants. This in turn activates detoxification at a cellular level. NRF2 also detoxifies the liver. From the first day I began taking it, thirty years of chronic fatigue stopped and at the time of writing it has now been close to two years! I wonder if my lifetime of ill-health was due to high levels of oxidative stress which my body, due to toxins or imbalances, had not been able to detoxify. Information or to purchase; dianneellis.com.au/contact

Redox signalling molecules
Within minutes of using redox signalling molecules I felt a nice tingling sensation in many areas of my body with a strange tightening then relaxation. Dr Gary Samuelson, an atomic medical physicist who worked to replicate and stabilize this product, explains that redox signalling molecules are a number of compounds produced by the mitochondria and act as either cellular messengers or cellular activators. They play a vital role in almost every function of our body, including repairing of cells, regenerating and replenishing, energy production, detoxification and activation of the immune system.

My grandfather died of cancer of the spine. When I had tearing feelings in my back and tingling in my feet, I suspected the same. Thermal imaging confirmed abnormalities through my spine, back, shoulders, and both breasts. Within a number of months after using redox signalling molecules I felt a profound strengthening in my back with less tearing and tingling sensations. The relief and gratitude were immense. Information or to purchase; dianneellis.com.au/contact

GcMAF
When I began using GcMAF I felt strong herxheimer reactions when my own immune system was activated and pathogens were being killed off. GcMAF is a protein our body makes which is found in high

levels in mammalian milk. It helps to upload Vit D and activate our macrophages, a type of white blood cell which is a vital part of our immune system. Many people are low in GcMAF.

7   Organic Essential Oils

When I was extremely ill my whole nervous system felt like it was on fire. I was overly sensitive to all stimulation both physical and emotional. Sounds, being touched and stress all triggered extreme discomfort in my body. Ylang Ylang oil rubbed on my ears provided a surprisingly high level of relief. It was only temporary but helpful each time. Peppermint oil capsules or a drop on my tongue dramatically eased digestive problems. Later, with severe spine troubles, peppermint oil down my spine was incredibly beneficial providing deep relaxation of the muscles and relief of pain. Some people may be sensitive to essential oils (see Eliminate Pathogens).
These can be bought at many outlets or contact me –
dianneellis.com.au/contact

8   Balance Biochemistry

A biomedical doctor can conduct a range of blood tests to see if you have any imbalances, genetic predispositions, toxins, pathogens etc that may be affecting your physical or emotional health. Specific treatment and supplementation can then be given. Many of these tests are specialised and not always available from every doctor (see Balance Biochemistry).

9   Dental

Hidden infections and toxic fillings can have a profound effect on our health. A simple filling gone wrong led to a dead tooth and hidden abscess which was poisoning my body. I had dramatic improvement when the tooth was removed (see Detox).

10   Love

The more love we feel within ourselves and have in our lives, the more happy hormones are released into our blood. Exercising, eating, meditation, sex, being in love, spiritual practices and connecting with nature can all produce endorphins, dopamine, serotonin, oxytocin and more. These happy hormones have been scientifically proven to regulate gene activity and create a healing response in our body (see Emotional and Soul Healing).

The Healing Journey

Biology and belief
While our genes are hereditary, so are many of the pathogens that are linked to many diseases and illnesses, and the underlying emotional patterns, conscious and subconscious thoughts and beliefs that are passed down through our families and loved ones.

Chronic Illness and herxheimer reactions
By the time a condition becomes chronic, parasites, viruses and bacteria have usually entered many parts of our body. There is often an accumulation of toxins and many systems within our body may not be functioning properly. Therefore, care must be taken not to overburden your body when you begin treating these conditions. Take time to allow your body to detoxify, readjust, recover and repair.

People with chronic illness must always start any new protocol slowly in case of a die off reaction when pathogens are killed and toxins are released. This reaction is called a herxheimer reaction and can be temporarily worse than the illness itself. When this happens it is recommend to lessen treatment or stop altogether and begin again at a slower pace when you feel better. It is essential to have a good detox programme (see Detox) in place to help your body to deal with the released toxins. I have found bicarb soda to be incredibly effective at reducing or stopping herx reactions.

Breakdown, repair and regenerate
It is extremely important to follow your instincts and tune in to what feels right for you. Once initial treatment has commenced, recovery from chronic illness can take time and adjustments to treatment protocols are often needed as time goes on. I was told that when using treatments for cancer those areas can become sensitive as the immune system goes to work and they break down. This is exactly what I experienced as areas of suspected cancer in my body became very tender. This at times may be confused with a problem in the body. I found I needed to allow this process of breakdown, repair and regeneration to unfold as my body was ready for it, taking higher doses when I felt up to it, and lessening or stopping until I felt ready for more. Seek professional support if you have concerns. Whether the feelings in your body are a natural healing process or a problem, never forget to tune in to your intuition as it is usually right.

Emotional connection

I was always a one pill wonder type of person. Just give me the medicine so I can get on with enjoying life. Until I became so dependent on more and more medication and eventually it didn't work anymore. I have discovered that when we clear the emotional connection to illness, health can be restored much more quickly. In acute or life-threatening situations there is no point looking for the emotional connection. Treatment has to be the priority. Once the situation is no longer serious, this is when the emotional connection to physical illness may present itself or be addressed if you choose to do so.

The underlying spiritual and emotional connection to all physical and mental dis-ease is not loving oneself fully.

Finding a deeper meaning?

Is there a message or something positive that can be found within your illness or negative experience? Is it possible you are carrying a burden of genetic memory passed down through the generations? Can your illness be alerting you to parts of yourself that have been hurt and closed down in defence? By listening to the messages of our body are we able to discover a deeper love within ourselves?

After a lifetime of chronic illness and suffering I can answer yes to all of the above. I have experienced all of these to be true. I've been on an incredible journey of healing, a journey I certainly would not have chosen to take, but what I have learnt and the strength I have gained has given me so much. I can't say I wouldn't take it all back, because I have been to the brink of death, to the darkest depths of my soul, and it was hell. A living hell that I never, ever want to experience again.

But by searching for a deeper meaning to it all, what I have found within this journey, within myself, is so very precious and wonderful. Illness has pushed me to let go of people or experiences that were not nurturing me. To face my fears and turn them into love. Instead of being filled with fear and struggle as I previously was, trying so hard to make life work, I now find life flowing so easily and effortlessly, filled with love and joy. I have learnt to love myself fully. At times I find myself walking around smiling, beaming with happiness and contentment, a contentment I never felt before.

My health is not yet one hundred percent, but I'm living a full and active life. Before I got Lyme disease I surrendered to chronic fatigue and living a limited life. I gave up my search for improved health. But now I may be healthier than many people who feel well, or think they have as much vitality as they can at their age, because I have found these incredible healing methods. But I know I can achieve even more so I won't limit myself. I strive to achieve higher levels of health and vibrance. For many years I had to be very careful due to the delicate state of my health, but slowly I began to feel the cause of my illnesses falling away. Step by step, I became stronger and healthier. Now, I can do more, lift more and surf more that I have in many years. I feel myself continuing to grow stronger every day. I have seen and spoken to many others who have had similar recoveries after thinking it was never possible. Believe me. It is possible.

The Whole Picture
Healing the physical body is so much more effective when combining methods for healing the whole self; mind, body and soul. My healing protocol combines all of the most effective and useful information I have gathered over my lifetime from many varying protocols and treatments. There are many places you will find much more information. I have just brought together what has been most effective for me. When I was gravely ill I kept thinking there must be someone or some health organisation who has the answers to the horrendous illness I was experiencing. Thankfully there was, but it wasn't just one answer or one resource.
I have discovered there are many doctors and researchers doing some brilliant work which has been extremely helpful, but unfortunately their work is not available through mainstream channels. It took me years to find the answers I needed and to put them all together in a way which worked for me. Some of these remedies are so simple and have been incredibly effective at helping me to regain health after nearly dying and being seriously ill for many years.
I have suffered with varying chronic and serious illnesses for most of my life, including chronic and severe asthma, allergies, recurrent sinus infections, headaches, digestive problems/IBS, chronic fatigue, post-traumatic stress disorder, depression, anxiety, early symptoms of multiple sclerosis, fibromyalgia symptoms, Lyme disease and suspected cancer throughout many areas of my body. I say suspected cancer because I chose not to have a biopsy or invasive testing.
Some experts believe puncturing a tumour or cancerous area can release cancerous cells into the blood stream which may then spread to other areas of the body. There are also reports that radiation used in testing can amplify problems. One of my doctors recommended thermal imaging

which confirmed areas of moderate level abnormalities in my back, spine, breasts, shoulders and neck, much of this on my right side leading down from a hidden tooth abscess. Thermal imaging also detected inflammation from partially dead teeth which did not show up as an obvious problem in x-rays. The worst of my trouble presented in my spine with pain and tearing sensations, accompanied with tingling in my hands and feet, and weakness and partial paralysis especially down my right side. For a few years I was very fearful of what was happening in my body but I kept going, searching and trying more and more remedies until I felt improvement in my overall health.

Testing

Although a correct diagnosis can be helpful, I was able to overcome serious life-threatening illness without knowing exactly what was wrong. When you activate your body's own self-healing mechanisms and your own body heals itself, it doesn't matter what was wrong. As long as you get better, that is the desired outcome. Seven years after being sent home from hospital, told I had anxiety when I was at deaths door, I finally had testing to confirm serious illness.

When testing for tick borne illnesses including Lyme disease, I used Australian Biologics in Sydney who have internationally recognised testing methods.

australianbiologics.com.au

Thermal imaging can detect changes in cells before a tumour develops, therefore it has been found to be more effective than mammograms. There are a number of thermography specialists in Australia and other countries.

goldcoastthermalimaging.com.au

Ultrasound has been recommended to me as a fairly safe alternative to potentially harmful testing methods such as x-rays and MRI. It seems counterproductive to use methods which potentially cause cancer to detect cancer. I would only use these methods if absolutely essential and as little as possible eg a dental x-ray before removal of a tooth. All doctors can give you a referral for an ultrasound.

Open your mind

'Be open to new learnings'. I realise how important that statement is in many ways for every individual on this earth. There are so many different options in health care. There are so many lessons and experiences available to us in life. Be open and inquisitive when a new way of thinking or an alternative treatment or remedy presents itself to you. It may just be beneficial.

During my lifetime with all the practitioners and experts I have been to and listened to, many have conflicting views and advice. Some criticise the work of others even when good results are achieved. There have been and continue to be so many new and incredible discoveries made every day, simplifying and/or revolutionising medicine. Many times I have been advised that a certain remedy is useless or even harmful, but it turned out to be very beneficial. We are all individual. Something may work well for one person but not for another.

We need to give people the freedom and respect to make their own informed choices of medical treatment. At the same time everyone needs to be wary of poor advice and con artists taking advantage of the vulnerable which can happen on all levels, from individual practitioners to large companies charading as respected health advisors. With overwhelming levels of illness in many societies around the world, individuals, practitioners, scientists, researchers and regulators need to accept and respect the work of genuine health professionals or pioneers who are having success for their patients without causing harm.

What should I do? How to take away the confusion.
There are so many possible options to take when you are not well. How do you know what is right for you? It would be ideal if we could follow one protocol set by experienced health professionals but due to the complexity of current health conditions and each person's individuality, treatment protocols are very dependent on the effectiveness and response from each individual.

After seeing as many practitioners as I could, with symptoms still remaining, I began to read and learn more about any treatment or remedy I was interested in or had been prescribed. I took advice from practitioners and listened to the feedback from other people. I began to develop an understanding of what was happening in my own body. I began to trust in my own common sense and intuition.

Introducing more unconventional treatments became confusing at times eg, bicarb, an antioxidant, cannot be taken with MMS, an oxidant, or the MMS will be negated. Probiotics cannot be taken at the same time as antimicrobials or the beneficial bacteria will be killed. I experimented to find what worked best for me. After a number of years taking many of these remedies, I knew very well the effects they would have on me and when the best time for me to take them was.

Early on, out of curiosity I began to use a pendulum, checking and cross checking the results. While I've been very sceptical of this in the past, I was quite surprised by the accuracy. I stated, 'My name is Dianne,' and the pendulum swung clockwise. I then stated 'My name is George,' and the pendulum swung back and forth. 'MMS1 is the best for me now.' The pendulum swung clockwise. 'MMS1 is not best for me now.' The pendulum swung back and forth. Time and time again when I tested and retested all the different remedies with the pendulum it gave me clear direction. Every day I checked and cross checked to confirm which remedies were best for me to take at that time.

Later I learned from someone to draw a large semicircle, similar to a protractor, on a piece of paper with lines numbered one to ten. Then, hold the pendulum at the centre point and when asking about a particular remedy or situation ask the question, 'How beneficial is this for me now?' followed by, 'How harmful is this?' I was shocked to discover how accurate this can be when the results coincided with all my experiences I'd had so far.

While I was amazed how the pendulum confirmed my choices, the most important thing to do is make sure you research, learn, and follow your own common sense and intuition about what treatments and remedies are right for you.

More on the underlying causes of disease and illness

Much of the latest research worldwide shows that most diseases and illnesses, including cancer, Lyme disease, neurological and autoimmune disorders are caused by toxins and/or pathogens; parasites, viruses and bacteria. This corresponds with my experiences. Parasites have been discovered inside cancerous cells, and once the parasites are killed the cells can repair or die off. Many people with multiple sclerosis, Alzheimer's, Parkinson's, autism, mental health problems and more, have had incredible recoveries when treating for Lyme disease caused by a bacterial infection.

Rather than just treating the pathogens, for full recovery we need to look at why our body was vulnerable to the pathogens. It doesn't matter what you are treating for, the same overall methods to truly recover health are the same. And that is exactly where the focus needs to be; not on overcoming the illness, but recovering overall health, for illness and disease cannot survive in a healthy body. Even if we do eliminate disease, if the body is not healthy, disease will usually return in one form or another.

I've had treatment in person, over the phone, and online with a huge number of local doctors and specialists, naturopaths and holistic practitioners, international doctors, energy healers and so called 'snake oil sellers'. I have used numerous protocols, eaten bugs and experimented with many gadgets, devices and seemingly toxic substances. I have followed the work of many doctors, specialists and researchers from around the world. I've spent six years participating in online support groups, every spare moment, often from daylight until after dark speaking to hundreds, thousands of unwell people. From all over the world, using all and more of the methods I list for nearly every disease or illness you can think of, they share their experiences, hardships, setbacks and successes. The underlying principle for successful recovery of their health is always the same whether treating for Lyme disease, cancer, allergies, digestive problems, neurological or autoimmune diseases, mental health conditions, chronic fatigue or anything else, despite whether or not they have even received a diagnosis.

What is the answer to good health?
The answer is getting rid of what is harming the body and the mind and replenishing what is needed. Simple right? Yes, it is simple but it can be hard work. If you have been unwell for a long time reversing the steps that led to chronic ill-health can be tedious and take time, precious time that you need to allow yourself. But the rewards are well worth it! For recovery of optimum health we need to commit fully to ourselves, body, mind and soul, from what we put into our body, to the way we think and what we believe. We also need to take a close look at the people and experiences we allow into our lives. I believe we can have good health instantaneously but it's letting go of old patterns that may not be nourishing us any longer that can be challenging. The ways we have lived our life, the food we eat, our thoughts and beliefs and our deep inner feelings.
Looking back over my life each different form of illness I've experienced has been successfully overcome using basically the same treatment principles:

- Cleanse and detox (including dental)
- Whole food diet
- Kill pathogens

- Replenish good gut bacteria
- Repair immune function
- Repair cell function
- Realign the body
- Balance biochemistry
- Harmonise the frequencies of the body
- Unlock the underlying emotional connection to physical illness and the corresponding cellular memory held in the body
- Connect to a higher love and oneness

Activate your body's own self-healing abilities
There is nothing more powerful than your own immune system. The intricate processes within our body interact with perfect precision. When this is disturbed, thrown out of balance and not functioning properly, disease states form. Many of the steps I share will help to restore health, but it is our own immune function that will ultimately enable us to regain and maintain good health.

Trust in your body
When you cut your finger how does it heal? It just does. Our body knows exactly what it needs to do to heal itself. It's just that we humans are destroying our external and internal environment. When you take away what is harming your body and give it what it needs, trust fully and wholly in your body's own ability to heal itself!

All in your head? The mind/body connection
The worst thing most patients with chronic illness hear is that it's all in their head. After years of undiagnosed chronic illness at times I was told it was simply anxiety. I spent many years exploring within myself to find how and when these conditions could have been created in my mind. After many years I finally received test results proving it wasn't all in my head and pathogens had been causing much of my ill-health over the years. In the meantime, I did find and release many underlying stresses that had left my immune system weakened and vulnerable to those conditions.
Each time I released a trauma or energy blockage within my body I found improvements, either due directly to the release of stress within my body, or thanks to a treatment or remedy that I would coincidently read or hear about which was particularly helpful for me at that time. This was

a seemingly miraculous process that occurred so many times I learnt not to question it, but simply to have faith in and appreciate it. My experience corresponded with Louise Hay's teachings that each illness has an underlying emotional connection, and it reaffirmed my belief in the words of many wise teachers who state that when we do the inner work the outside world will follow suit.

This is not to lessen for one moment the severity of some physical conditions and their absolute need for medical or natural treatment. I know people who have had miraculous healings, including a good friend of mine who had relief from serious, long term chronic illness due to Lyme disease and tick-borne infections, after receiving reconnective healing. While I have wished so many times to have this type of experience I have come to the conclusion my need for physical remedies has helped me to become grounded and centred within my body which I have found difficult to do most of my life. I also suspect I needed to do the hard yards to clear so much of the pain I carried, which actually became a blessing, enabling me to reach deeper levels of love than I had ever experienced before. Nonetheless I believe energy medicine and the power of our mind should never be underestimated.

Do you give away your energy, your life force?
While much of the latest research shows that parasites are an underlying cause of most diseases and illness, Louise Hay suggests that parasites in our body represent giving away our power to others. Therefore, the people, past and present, that we have in our lives, and our conscious and/or subconscious thoughts, beliefs and feelings about these relationships, has a direct and significant effect on our health or ill-health. This coincides with the work of Dr Klinghardt who insists that psychological work is a vital part of health recovery, emphasising that addressing parasites needs to be a priority for all chronic conditions.

Dr Klinghardt has found big emotional shifts occur when we cleanse parasites from our body and we need to be prepared for the possible release of long held traumas or emotional hurts when doing so. Although this concept may be new to some, just being aware of it may be beneficial to understand some of the experiences you have before, during or after treatment. I had this experience during liver cleansing but didn't realise the connection at the time. Due to traumatic events in my early life I had done a lot of counselling and breathwork before I became seriously ill with Lyme disease. This helped me to deal with the experiences that were arising. I was also very aware of the effect my feelings about the relationships with people in my life, past and present, had on my physical body. I have no doubt this is a very significant key in our recovery from chronic illness.

Take control of your health
While the basic principle to health recovery is the same, I don't know one person who has had identical treatment to another. There are always variables to consider such as what we eat, the exercise we do, our individual biochemistry and the different practitioners, medications and treatments we have access to and so on. One treatment for parasites might not go well for one person but is perfectly suited to another. At times two highly regarded practitioners may provide you with conflicting advice. Therefore, it is very important for each of us to work out what is working well for us. Study, research and speak to others who have had the condition you are experiencing. If you are able to, seek out a team of good practitioners you feel confident with and don't hesitate to obtain a second, third or twentieth opinion.
If you begin a treatment and it isn't working for you, be open to investigating why that might be. Are you taking the correct dose? Maybe you are having a herxheimer reaction, which often occurs before improvement. Talk to your practitioner. Unfortunately sometimes due to the intensity of some illnesses people find it difficult to receive enough practitioner support. This is where online support groups can play a vital role. If you feel something isn't right always listen to that voice within. Is the alarm going off for fear of uncertainty, or is there a genuine reason for you to be concerned and a change in your course of action is required? It would be very easy if we could just go to a doctor, take a pill and be done with it. With the complex conditions occurring in current times, recovery of optimum health usually takes a little more than that, but it is very achievable. I have spoken to people in wheel chairs with multiple sclerosis and mothers of severely autistic children who have experienced huge recoveries by taking control of their health and following the basic principles that I discuss here.

What to do if you are bitten by a tick, suspect Lyme disease or have symptoms of any disease or illness which is mimicked by Lyme disease?
If you are bitten by a tick, even if you don't have any symptoms, many forms of bacteria can lay dormant within the body for years so it is strongly recommended to take preventative action. Lyme disease can become serious and life-threatening. When treated early within the first

6-8 weeks treatment can be very successful. Left untreated it can become chronic and very difficult to treat. Unfortunately, most health departments in many countries don't provide adequate treatment for Lyme disease or tick-borne illness and suggest that Post Lyme Disease Syndrome is the cause of on-going symptoms when they are unable to treat it properly. This belief has been ridiculed by Lyme specialists and patients.

I found a Lyme specialist online in America who is a molecular biologist, herbalist, homeopath and nutritionist which I found very helpful. There are very few medical or natural health professionals in Australia who are knowledgeable enough to treat Lyme disease, Lyme-like or tick-borne Illness effectively. Even if they are up to date with the latest protocols, unfortunately, doctors may not be able to provide that treatment due to regulations on treating Lyme disease. In Australia a number of doctors have had their licence restricted for doing so.

The Lyme Disease Association of Australia have a comprehensive data base of information about Lyme disease and tick-borne illness, including recommended treatment protocols, Lyme literate practitioners, and the current medical and political stance in Australia. The Karl McManus Foundation is also dedicated to prevention and treatment in Australia. Many countries have Lyme disease organisations providing similar information in their country which can usually be found easily online.

Australia - lymedisease.org.au   karlmcmanus.org.au   ticna.org.au
America - lymedisease.org   UK - lymediseaseuk.com

Lyme literate doctors
Many Lyme literate doctors and associations who are knowledgeable about treating Lyme disease will recommend six weeks of antibiotics, after receiving a tick bite. If you have a chronic condition, long-term antibiotics may be recommended. Short and long-term antibiotics can have mild to severe side effects. Some holistic Lyme literate doctors may recommend natural alternatives which can be very powerful or a combination of both.

Mainstream medicine
Some people who are bitten by a tick and present to a doctor in Australia are given the recommended 6 weeks antibiotics. Unfortunately, most people report being sent home with inadequate treatment. The health department in Australia, at the time of writing this book, does not recognise Lyme disease therefore treatment is not readily available. In

fact many doctors have been reprimanded for using unconventional treatments, which are commonly used overseas, to address the symptoms of Lyme disease.

Overseas clinics
There are numerous clinics around the world, such as in Germany and Cypress, which provide specialised treatment for Lyme disease using many natural and advanced treatments. Occasionally some people don't have good results but most people have improvement.

Natural approach
There are many natural remedies and treatments which are used to kill bacteria that may have been transmitted by a tick including:

- Essential oils
- Herbal tinctures
- Homeopathics
- Silvercillin/colloidal silver
- MMS1/CD, MMS2
- Redox signalling molecules
- AmpCoil
- Rife / Dr Clark Zappper
- Bioresonance
- Hyperthermia
- Ozone treatment

My preferred treatment if bitten by a tick
If I am bitten by a tick I always use MMS and I may use one or a number of the following as well:

- MMS1/CD and MMS2 following Jim Humble's protocols
- Essential oils
- Colloidal silver
- Antimicrobial herbs especially Dr Klinghardt's Lyme Cocktail
- Homeopathics
- AmpCoil

jimhumble.is   Lyme Cocktail - sophiaeducate.com
ampcoil.com

Extensive Protocol ... Recovery of Optimum Health

With incredible advances in modern technology and research methods, new medical discoveries are being made all the time. Therefore, the protocols I have used are always open to change depending on new advancements in treatments and their outcomes. I have listed almost every remedy I have used but not all that have been prescribed by complimentary doctors or the molecular biologist who treated me. This is purely because the information is very complex and I do not feel confident with my knowledge to share all those details.

The basic principles to health recovery always remain the same - remove what is harming your body and replenish what is needed. Below are the steps towards health recovery that I have found to be the most effective in order of importance and accessibility. You can immediately change what you put into your mouth, what you think, and what food you buy from the shops. It is also very important to get the detoxification pathways and self-healing mechanisms in your body working as soon as possible, hence the order of steps I list here:

1. Detoxification
2. Stress release and positive intention
3. Diet/Gut health
4. Alkalize your body
5. Activate your body's self-healing mechanisms
6. Eliminate pathogens - parasites, viruses, bacteria and mould
7. Balance biochemistry
8. Realign your body
9. Exercise
10. Energy Healing
11. Emotional Healing
12. Soul Healing

1 Detox

Kidney and liver cleansing
The most important step before commencing any treatment or protocol is cleansing our two main filtering organs. Many processed unnatural foods are hard for our body to digest and can lead to congestion in all areas of our body. Parasites and toxins can also create blockages. We change the filters in our cars and appliances regularly but rarely cleanse the filters of our body. Imagine if your sewerage pipes blocked up, what a mess there would be. This is what happens in our body which needs to deal with excess waste which is not being filtered properly when our kidneys and liver are congested.

While there are many methods to detoxify the body, cleansing these two major organs is a vital first step. There is no doubt simple liver cleansing saved my life. It is recommended to commence a kidney cleanse before the liver cleanse so the kidneys can be prepared and ready to handle what is released by the liver. I was given Juniper berry tea for one day to cleanse my kidneys but I was in such a serious condition my naturopath put me straight onto the liver cleanse. My health was deteriorating so quickly I have no doubt this was a wise step for me and saved my life. Many kidney and liver cleansing herbs can be bought over the counter at health food stores, herbal dispensaries or online. Tinctures are also available and can be stronger than teas. I have been happy to stay with the warm, soothing effect of the teas rather than tinctures which was recommended by one of my practitioners. I was instructed to take one teaspoon of one herb, or a mixture of herbs, half hour before breakfast and dinner.

drclark.net
liverdoctor.com
mullumherbals.com.au
gardenofedenorganics.net.au

Kidney cleanse
The kidneys filter our blood to produce urine composed of extra fluid and waste products. They work to balance sodium and water, acidity and alkalinity. The kidneys play a vital role in removing heavy metals. There are many herbal teas for kidney cleansing such as:

- Juniper berry
- Hydrangea
- Gravel root
- Marshmallow
- Goldenrod
- Ginger
- Parsley

Liver Cleanse
The liver is one of the most important organs in our body. It filters our blood removing parasites, viruses, bacteria, dead cells, cancer cells and toxins. If the liver becomes congested many of these substances recirculate throughout our body having a detrimental effect on every system. When using treatments to kill parasites, viruses and bacteria, liver cleansing is a vital step to remove these pathogens and the resulting toxins and to minimise 'herxeimer' reactions.

I cannot repeat it enough; liver cleansing was the most valuable and effective method to improve my health when I was seriously ill. There is no doubt that just one simple mug of alfalfa leaf tea morning and night saved my life. Within one day the area of my liver felt very swollen as though I had a football under my ribs. Later that day I went to the toilet and knew my liver was flushing out. From then on my health slowly began to improve. After a number of months I realised all my food allergies were gone. I use a number of herbal teas for cleansing the liver daily such as:

- Alfalfa leaf
- Dandelion leaf
- St Mary's thistle
- Liquorice root
- Skullcap
- Peppermint
- Fresh lemon and ginger

Dental Cleanse
Bacteria and hidden infections such as those beneath root canals and dead teeth have been linked to cancer and serious heart conditions. The bacteria from these dead teeth goes directly into the blood stream potentially poisoning the whole body. As my dentist says, most people with amalgam fillings will have a mouth that is shut down by workplace

health and safety. Amalgam fillings release heavy metals, mercury being the most toxic. Removal of these fillings is recommended, but must be done with extreme caution by a highly trained dentist using specifically designed safety methods to prevent mercury poisoning. Protective methods used will be a rubber dam to prevent any filling material falling down the throat, separate oxygen supply, and very high speed suction to remove filling material and the air around it while drilling occurs. Unsafe removal of amalgam fillings can result in serious heavy metal/mercury toxicity.

Removal of amalgam fillings and dead teeth can be a big shock to the body. When I was seriously ill I know my body would not have handled the procedure of either. I had done a lot of liver and kidney cleansing with the herbal teas when I discovered a hidden abscess and subsequent removal of the tooth enabled significant improvement in my health. Thankfully my amalgam fillings had been safely removed many years before.

Since finishing part 1 of this book, I rubbed the redox gel on the gum of a tooth I had been suspicious of for a long time, but was avoiding losing any more teeth. Later I felt tenderness and a slight shooting pain. Immediately I was sure there must be a problem. Thermal imaging confirmed inflammation feeding down my throat in the area of two teeth which didn't show obvious problems on an x-ray. While I avoid x-rays my dentist does recommend an OPG before any major procedure. He did a cold test on all my teeth and detected one that was unresponsive, meaning the nerve was dead, and one which was over-responsive, which is often due to one or more dead nerves in the molar making the other nerve/s extra sensitive. Due to my health history, I insisted on removal of both teeth which were confirmed to be almost all dead but one nerve.

Hal Huggins - hugginsappliedhealing.com

Heavy metals
The harmful effects of heavy metals on the body are well documented and are proving to have a much bigger link to disease and illness than first recognised. Heavy metals are everywhere in our environment and are found in our air, food, water, medications, tooth fillings and can be held in every area of the body with potentially detrimental effects to every system of the body.

There are a number of methods recommended to remove heavy metals from our body. These are called chelators. I have used:

- MMS1/CD
- Homeopathics
- Cilantro
- Spirulina
- Chlorella
- Diatomaceous earth
- Activated charcoal
- Bentonite clay
- AmpCoil

Also highly recommended are:
- High silicon mineral water
- Ionic foot spa
- DMPS

Binders
When detoxing heavy metals it's important to use binders. When taken internally these substances will bind to toxins and heavy metals in our body enabling them to be more easily eliminated and prevent reabsorption into the body. A binder will help to excrete heavy metals through the gastrointestinal system in the faeces rather than via the kidneys, therefore having a protective action:

- Cilantro
- Spirulina
- Chlorella
- Diatomaceous earth
- Activated charcoal
- Bentonite clay

Kerri Rivera recommends MMS1/CD to neutralize heavy metals. It seems that aluminium is one of the metals causing the most health concerns at present. Professor Christopher Exley shares the simple method of drinking mineral water high in silicic acid, the biologically available form of silicon, to easily rid the body of aluminium. He demonstrates in his research that aluminium comes out of the body with silicon in the urine along with other metals. Dr Klinghardt highly recommends ionic foot spas explaining that during an ion cleanse detox foot bath session, large concentrations of negative hydrogen ions are released during the process of electrolysis. These ions are absorbed into the body by osmosis through the epidermis of the foot. Once entered into the system, these negatively charged ions act as an ultra-high powered antioxidant.

There are many chelating agents to draw heavy metals out of the body, but this needs to be done carefully because if the metals are not released from the body straight away, they can be redeposited in other areas causing more harm. Dr Klinghardt states that supporting the kidneys to remove these metals from the body is the safest way to do so. He says DMPS is a powerful method to assist the kidneys to release heavy metals. DMPS (Sodium 2,3-dimercaptopropane-l-sulfonate) is a sulfonic acid salt that forms complexes with heavy metals such as mercury, cadmium, arsenic, lead, copper, silver, tin, and others. It was first developed in China then introduced to Russia to be used for workers injured by exposure to heavy metals. DMPS is best used under the guidance of a health practitioner. It is recommended to have amalgam fillings safely removed before some heavy metal detoxification processes such as the use of DMPS as it may draw the metals out of the fillings.

Strangely, as stated below in the parasite section, Dr Klinghardt finds that some parasites can have a positive effect on our body by up taking heavy metals and therefore lessening the load on our systems. Thus, it is very important to have a detox program in place before killing parasites.

Kerri Rivera – www.ketokerri.com
Dr Klinghardt - sophiaeducate.com

Mould

Mould toxins can have severe and debilitating effects on our body; therefore it is highly recommended to treat mould in and outside of the body. Any other steps to regain health will be hampered until this is addressed. There are many different treatments for mould including:

- MMS1/CD
- Bicarb Soda
- Bentonite clay
- Probiotics/fermented foods
- Ginger
- Garlic

- Goldenseal
- Cayenne
- Activated Charcoal
- Chlorophyll
- Essential oils including Eucalyptus, Tea Tree, Sage,
- Thyme, Clove, Cinnamon

Jim Humble states that while MMS can treat some mould, it is not always effective. In this case he recommends bentonite clay. The essential oils listed are some of the most popular for mould but many have anti-fungal properties. In the home bicarb soda, vinegar, hydrogen peroxide and/or an essential oil diffuser work well.

Liver flush
When I was seriously ill there is no way my body would have handled the liver flush process. I used the gentle liver cleansing herbal teas for eighteen months before learning about this method. I completed the Dr Hulda Clark liver flush many times and was astounded with the results. This process uses a recipe of epsom salts, olive oil and grapefruit juice to flush stones, parasites, toxins and congestion out of the liver. It is quite an intense and at times uncomfortable process. I have spoken to people who have had great success with the flush and two or three people who were very ill. It seems the people who were ill unfortunately did not carry out the parasite and kidney cleanses which Dr Clark insists must be undertaken before commencing the flush. I think it is also a good idea to do the more gentle liver cleansing teas before the flush.

After feeling improvements and having exhausted all other treatment options available to me, following directions strictly, I completed twenty-three flushes during eighteen months with no trouble apart from some temporary nausea. I removed over 1000 stones during this period and felt improvements in my health each time. Some stones were partially calcified but most were not, these being called cholesterol stones. Dr Clark believes we all have congestion in our liver and up to two thousand stones which can be cleared using the liver flush. This may remedy many health conditions including food allergies.

I have since learnt about methods to dissolve stones such as consuming large amounts of apple juice. Also essential oils, being natural plant terpenes, have been used. I believe these combined with liver cleansing herbs and enemas or colonics may be very effective. I am sure the flush

removed many parasites and toxins from my body as well as stones and due to the very noticeable improvements in my health, I believe it is a very valuable process. This type of liver flush is recommended as a vital part in a number of cancer protocols such as 'The Perfect Storm Cancer Protocol'.
drclark.net
cancertutor.com/perfect_storm

Salt water flush
A salt water flush is a good way of cleaning out your whole digestive tract, especially the colon. It is recommended to drink a mixture of two teaspoons of pure sea salt in one litre of water, adding lemon if desired. First thing in the morning before eating is preferable or at least an hour or two after. I came across the salt water flush when researching more about Kerri Rivera's recommendation to drink ocean water for replacement of minerals as mentioned in her MMS1/CD protocol. Kerri's advice to mix purified water with ocean water prevents loose motions and allows the salt water with all its mineral to be absorbed into the body. I drink ocean water each day and occasionally I drink it pure as a salt water flush.

Enemas and colonics
Enemas and colonics are very effective at cleansing the bowel of parasites and waste material, including build-up of waste on the bowel walls. Coffee enemas have a strong detoxifying effect on the liver and bile ducts. MMS1/CD enemas will kill many parasites, viruses and bacteria in the bowel. I have done water, coffee and MMS1/CD enemas. They all seemed to be helpful to a degree also.

Fasting
There are many types of fasting people carry out such as juice and water fasting where their dietary intake is just that; juice or water. There are some reports of people having great success and their immune system being repaired within days. Fasting can activate a state of autophagy and mitophagy. Autophagy is where the body will consume its own tissue, particularly damaged or cancerous cells. Mitophagy is when damaged mitochondria are removed from the cell via autophagy. Dr Joseph Mercola highly recommends fasting, and intermittent fasting, alternating with times of feasting. He acknowledges there can be side effects and it's not suitable for everyone.

From my experience of fasting, I believe when our body is already in a high state of stress it can send the signal that something is wrong, therefore the body's processes may be disrupted even more. Also, pathogens in the body that are used to being fed regularly will get, as Kerri Rivera calls it, POWS; pissed off worm syndrome. I have spoken to a couple of people who have had disastrous results, most likely due to pushing themselves too hard in this process.

But, when we are ready and able to, I have no doubt fasting will accelerate our body's healing processes. For a long time I felt very unwell if I missed meals and realised my body would not cope with any fasting. When my body become stronger I began intermittent short term fasting by simply missing breakfast. As my tolerance to fasting grew I also began to miss lunch; therefore fasting throughout the day. I maintained remedies to kill off pathogens and activate my immune system and felt them working more effectively while fasting. I also noticed benefits to my digestion.

Now I only fast when it's convenient and if I don't have a busy day ahead. I believe I can feel the benefits Dr Mercola describes as my body has the opportunity to clear out toxins and dead cells, repair and rejuvenate. If you attempt fasting, be strong in your conviction to give it a go but don't push yourself to a point of harm. Try small steps. Listen to your body. Be gentle with yourself.

mercola.com

Juicing
There are many wonderful benefits to juicing, the obvious being the immediate availability of high level nutrients into our body. This can give our cells, organs and all the systems in our body a boost. There are some beliefs that consuming juice without the fibre of the fruit or vegetable can be excessive for our body. Research this topic and do what feels right for you.

2 Stress Release and Positive Intention

In this moment before we have the time to go and see a practitioner, buy a remedy or put food in our mouths, we have the ability to immediately change our thoughts and beliefs. As cell biologist Dr Bruce Lipton states, every thought we have has an effect on our body. If we have stressful thoughts, stress hormones are immediately released into our blood. If we have happy thoughts, happy hormones are released. Every cell in our body responds to these hormones. Muscle tension and restriction of blood flow may result. All bodily and cell functions can be impacted.

Even if you are terrified by a condition you may be experiencing in your body, simply by stating to yourself a few times, 'I am safe', your body will settle to a degree on some level, even if you are not aware of it. It's also very important to set intentions to let go of painful situations and dis-ease from the body, with ease. To the best of our ability, opening to and filling ourselves with love is one of the easiest, most effective ways to do this.

Regulating breathing patterns, taking nice full relaxed breaths into your belly, putting your hand on your heart and thinking loving thoughts can shift the heart into a smooth, flowing rhythm. When we are able to shift into this coherent mode, many changes occur in our body. On a neurological level the heart and brain become more synchronised, neurons in the brain operate at a higher level of efficiency, hormones throughout the body become more balanced, cognitive functions are enhanced, short and long term memory improve, and our ability to focus and make decisions is enhanced.

It is well documented that stress is one of the biggest underlying causes of ill-health. Many diseases and illnesses are triggered by emotional and/or physical stress. In acute situations, addressing only the stress caused by that condition is a priority. If a condition becomes chronic, addressing the long term underlying stress or anxiety that may have left the immune system more vulnerable to that condition is recommended.

heartmath.com

3 Diet/Gut health

If we are unwell we have the ability to make an immediate improvement in our health simply by controlling what we put into our mouth. Nothing is better than a diet of fresh whole fruit, vegetables and protein. Many accredited doctors who have great success with their patients recommend ketogenic or paleo diets, preferably organic. Many doctors highly recommend a ketogenic diet which contains a high consumption of healthy fats, moderate intake of high-quality protein and minimal amounts of carbohydrates with little or no grains. This type of diet will induce our body into a state of nutritional ketosis so we burn fat instead of carbohydrates which is our body's preferred source of fuel.

Dr Joseph Mercola recommends cycling in and out of a ketogenic diet and combining intermittent fasting which has shown to provide significant health benefits, including decreased risk of cancer and inflammation, improved muscle mass, lower insulin levels, improved mental capacity and increased longevity. Dr Mercola also believes cycling between feast and famine is very beneficial. Fasting upregulates autophagy and mitophagy which are the natural cleansing processes necessary for optimal cellular renewal and function. Stem cells are activated and mitochondrial biosynthesis stimulated. During the feasting stage when carbohydrates are increased rejuvenation processes take place.

I have been vegan and vegetarian at times due to my previous allergy to dairy and my spiritual and animal welfare beliefs, but felt very weak and struggled greatly. I noticed huge improvement in my health and reduction of Lyme symptoms when I stopped eating grains or any processed food and ate only whole foods such as vegetables, meat, fish, eggs, healthy fats and fruit. Of course some individual's needs may vary, and vegetarians may choose alternatives.

thepaleoway.com

Stop feeding disease and illness
Underlying many diseases and illnesses are pathogens. Many of these pathogens thrive on grains and sugars which also create an acidic environment within our body allowing the bad bugs to thrive even more. Removing all processed and sugary foods from your diet and eating whole fresh food creates an environment which is less conducive to pathogens will have an immediate, positive effect on your health.

Replenish
Replenishing the vitamins, minerals and good bacteria in our body is a vital step towards regaining health. Harmful bacteria, viruses and parasites deplete our body of these crucial substances. I have taken many processed supplements but now find the simple steps below, combined with any supplements recommended by my biomedical doctor, to be ample. See Balance Biochemistry section below. Be wary of taking too many supplements that may not be correct for your biochemistry. They may also contain 'fillers', congest the liver and could do more harm than good.

Probiotics
While it is vital to rid our body of harmful bacteria, good bacteria are essential to our health. Bacterial cells are much smaller than our own cells but incredibly there are more of them in our body than our own cells. Much of our digestive system is comprised of good bacteria, often referred to as microbiome, which plays a huge role in the digestion and absorption of our food and nutrients. It plays a large role in activating and deactivating genes, breaking down food, enhancing the immune system and even produces serotonin, a happy brain hormone. Introducing probiotics to your diet can be commenced as soon as possible. I must say though, I have noticed a very significant activation in my immune system often when taking fermented foods, which can at times be too strong. This has particularly happened when taking homemade GcMAF using milk kefir, so if you are chronically ill taking small amounts to start with is good. I make my own probiotics including:

- Fermented vegetables
- Water kefir
- Milk kefir
- Kombucha

When I began making and ingesting my own fermented foods, to my surprise I had a significant improvement in my health and weight. Fermented vegetables and kefir contain much higher concentrations of beneficial bacteria than most probiotic supplements, the bacteria are active and the fermentation process predigests the food which is filled with vital nutrients, minerals, enzymes and amino acids.
Donna Gates bodyecology.com

Water
It is important to drink at least 2-3 litres of clean water a day. Not only is that our daily requirement for optimal function, being well hydrated will help our body to detoxify especially when we are undertaking cleanses.

Water purification
Most water supplies throughout many countries are either contaminated with toxins, pollutants or pathogens. A lot of treated water has been found to contains chemicals which have been linked to cancer. A good filter can remove most of these unwanted substances. As recommended by Jim Humble I use MMS1/CD to purify water especially when travelling.
www.clarencewaterfilters.com.au
www.mmsaustralia.com.au (HCL-MMS1 Convenience Pack)

Ocean water
To replace minerals in the body, Kerri Rivera highly recommends drinking ocean water, the natural minerals of the earth, which we are able to easily absorb and contains ninety minerals which is the entire periodic table. We need minerals especially in any detoxification protocol. Ocean water also revitalizes our cells and provides conductivity in the brain. In her CD protocol Kerri recommends drinking ocean water up to tolerance, even up to one cup per day for adults.
Though I live near the beach and spend a lot of time in the ocean I did not take this step for a very long time, purely from lack of interest. That was a big mistake! Since taking ocean water each day, I have noticed huge improvements in my energy and feelings of wellbeing. On occasions I have run out and missed it for a couple of days and begin wondering why I am not feeling as well as I had been! It seems ocean water has all the minerals at the correct ratios/levels that we need. It is in fact almost identical to human blood. If you do not have a clean supply of ocean water or if you live inland there are packaged options and salt protocols available and worth looking into.
Since discovering benefits of fulvic-humic acid, Kerri has updated her protocol to include this as a powerful mineral supplement.

Ayurvedic principles
We all have an individual constitution, some of us being naturally slender and light, or strong and sturdy, a tendency to be hot or cold, patient or fiery. These are all qualities attributed to differing types of constitutions, also called Doshas as recognised in Ayurveda as Vata, Pitta and Kapha.

Each Dosha is a combination of two of the elements. Kapha is water and earth. Vata is a combination of ether and air. Pitta is fire and water.

When a Dosha becomes excessive we can become out of balance physically, emotionally and mentally. While these ayurvedic principles are relevant to all areas of our lives, I found them particularly helpful with my diet.

Finding out which Dosha you are can help you to make simple but important changes in your dietary and lifestyle choices to help your whole system stay in balance. When I was told I was predominately Vata and cooked foods would be more beneficial for me, I put on some weight and felt stronger. I had been eating cooked foods for breakfast and dinner but cutting down salads for lunch and adding more cooked food made a big difference. Someone who is Pitta and has more heat in their body will do better with cooling foods such as salads. It is likely you can determine which Dosha you are by learning about each of their qualities. Seeing an Ayurvedic practitioner is beneficial.

Jacinta McEwen - omhealing.com.au

4 Alkalize Your Body

Bicarb Soda

Bicarb soda was a game changer for me. It provided huge relief of horrendous Lyme symptoms and it is very easy to access. If our body is too acidic it can be detrimental to every system in our body. For our everyday survival our blood pH level needs to be between 7.35 and 7.45. When acid levels are too high our body will rob alkaline minerals from our bones and organs to help neutralize acids which can lead to weakened organs and osteoporosis. Calcium can build up as arthritis. There are many diets and methods to alkalize the body. Most of us eat a diet or grew up with a diet which promotes an acidic environment in our body. This can be difficult to reverse using diet alone. Pathogens that cause disease and illness thrive in an acidic environment but cannot survive in an alkaline environment.

Taking one teaspoon of bicarb soda dissolved in a glass of water four times a day, half hour before or one and a half hours after meals gave me almost immediate relief of Lyme symptoms including muscle pain, cramping, tingling, severe anxiety, and herxheimer reactions. Spraying a dilution on my skin also provided immediate relief from many Lyme disease symptoms. My body felt much more relaxed and I was able to sleep much better. In fact I felt so much relief, for six months this was the only remedy I used. I felt the bicarb working in the areas of suspected cancer, and my next six month thermal imaging showed some areas of improvement and some areas of resolution.

I have spoken to many people with different conditions taking bicarb and most seem to notice either small or dramatic improvements. It is advised there may be slight side effects, which are symptoms of detoxification, and some people may experience pain when arthritis or damaged areas of the body break down. This has been the case with a number of people I have spoken to but lowering the dose to allow the process to occur at a slower rate as recommended does provide relief. I have not heard of anyone having herxheimer reactions from taking bicarb soda.

There are beliefs that bicarb should not be taken due to reduction in stomach acid which may interfere with digestion. Despite this, due to the incredible relief of daily agonizing symptoms I would certainly be placing it on the top of the list, particularly for fast accessible relief of Lyme symptoms.

I buy from a health shop or <u>safesoda.com.au</u>

Hydrogen Water
Hydrogen water is becoming very popular as an antioxidant and a powerful way to alkalise the body. Many alkalizing waters only buffer acidity without removing it. However Kerri Rivera has developed **Hydroxide Water™** from limestone which has a powerful alkalising effect without being detrimental to stomach acid.

Kerri believes bicarb soda interferes with stomach acid levels disrupting digestion too much so she uses what she calls Hydroxide Water™ developed from food grade calcium hydroxide, which is limestone.

"Interestingly, although water is made up of two hydrogen protons and one oxygen proton, when it splits apart it always splits into one hydrogen proton, and a hydrogen proton and an oxygen proton remain together," Kerri explains. "The hydrogen proton and oxygen proton that remain together are called hydroxide (OH−). Hydrogen protons and hydroxide ions do not like being separated and a strong electro-magnetic bond attracts them to each other. When hydroxide is introduced into an environment where excess acidity exists, it immediately seeks out the hydrogen protons to combine with them and become water. This is why hydroxide is such a strong acid eliminator. This results in hydration of the body with the creation of more water molecules. Inflammation is reduced. Detoxification, energy and oxygen levels are increased."

On the day I planned to send this book to the printers I happened to meet a Chinese doctor who makes **hydrogen water** in a specific way to ensure high enough levels of hydrogen to effectively alkalise the body. Although I only had the chance to try two cans before sending this book to print I did notice an effect in my body. Due to this fortuitous meeting I believe his Opal water is certainly meant to be shared.

I have not tried Kerri's Hydoxide water but have no doubt it is good.
ketokerri.com
opalwater.com.au

5 Activate Your Body's Own Self-Healing Mechanisms

Circadian Rhythm and Sleep
Our internal body clock, or circadian rhythm is a twenty four hour cycle particularly affecting our sleeping, waking and eating patterns. It is influenced by stimulation from our environment such as sunlight, temperature, the food and times of day that we eat. In response to this stimuli, signals are sent to the hypothalamus which governs the circadian rhythm and produces hormones such as melatonin, which causes sleepiness. Many of our biological and psychological processes are governed by our circadian rhythm. This is why it is very important to have good amounts of quality sleep every day and regular routines.

Nutrigenomics/Biohacking, NRF2
Nutrigenomics is the study of how nutrition can affect our genes. I didn't know much about this topic but learnt very quickly due to the dramatic improvement in my health that NRF2 provided. Dr Joe McCord was the first doctor to discover oxidative stress in the body and its connection to nearly all disease, illness and injury. One molecule of Vitamin C will remove one free radical in our body, while one molecule of our own powerful antioxidants will remove one million. So Dr McCord worked with a team of doctors to find something to activate our body's own antioxidants; glutathione, superoxide dismutase and catalase. They found that a specific combination of five herbs, turmeric, milk thistle, green tea, bacoba and ashwaganda, will activate the release of the NRF2 protein in our cells, which in turn signals our genes to produce more of our own antioxidants. In the last five years Dr McCord has discovered that not only is NRF2 activating the genes which produce our own antioxidants, it's also having a positive effect on over four to five hundred other genes. He explains that it upregulates the genes that help our cells survive and decreases the genes that are doing damage and causing problems.
I was very sceptical that this seemingly simple combination of herbs could have such a profound effect on people's health until I experienced it myself. I then spoke to others who gained relief from back pain, arthritis, depression, fatigue, lung disorders, eczema, learning disorders and much more.
A combination of Acetyl L-Carnitine, Coenzyme Q10, Alpha-lipoic acid, Grape Extract and Quercetin, has also been developed to activate the

NRF1 pathway in our cells. This helps to repair and increase production of mitochondria which are the energy systems of our cells. Most disease and illness is linked to mitochondria dysfunction, therefore keeping these little powerhouses healthy is vitally important.
dianneellis.com.au/nrf2

Redox signalling molecules
Redox signalling molecules are a number of compounds produced by the mitochondria and act as either cellular messengers or cellular activators. They play a vital role in almost every function of our body, including repairing of cells, regenerating and replenishing, energy production, detoxification and activation of the immune system. They also give our cells the messages to kill pathogens and protect against parasites, viruses and bacteria.

Dr Gary Samuelson, an atomic medical physicist, has found a way to replicate identically and stabilise redox signalling molecules in a safe bio-compatible salt water solution and in gel form. He talks about its ability to flip the genetic switches that help the cells to rebalance when there has been damage. Hearing Dr Samuelson discuss how the action of the redox signalling molecules, which are reactive oxygen species, ties in with the oxidation mechanisms by which MMS1/CD works fascinated me. It also confused me a little because for many years we've all heard a lot about the harmful effects of oxidation and the powerful benefits of antioxidants. Dr Samuelson explains it is vital for us to have a balance of both.

Many people report improvement from almost all health conditions from immune and digestive disorders, autism and Lyme disease to cancer, head injuries and more. The redox gel has received praise for clearing up skin conditions and for cosmetic purposes. Although I have given little thought to skin enhancing cosmetic processes in the past, having been a surfer, as I age I am now appreciating all of the properties of this gel.

I have experienced huge levels of improvement in the areas of suspected cancer in my back since applying the redox molecules. So much so that I believe Dr Samuelson's comment that 'redox signalling molecules are the biggest breakthrough since penicillin' is very true. A friend of mine who had cancer has a naturopath who sent away for blood tests on several cancer patients, all with differing cancers. These tests were to determine which treatment out of all remedies available, mainstream or holistic, would be most effective for each form of cancer. She was astounded to

learn the redox products came out on top of the list for every form of cancer.
dianneellis.com.au/redox-signalling-molecules

GcMAF
GcMAF can immediately activate our immune system to kill pathogens and clear out damaged and cancerous cells. A protein in our body, GcMaf is a vital part of our immune system which uploads vitamin D to activate macrophages, a form of white blood cells. Most of us are lacking GcMAF and without it our immune system is disabled. Many people have high levels of nagalase which depletes our body's own GcMAF. Supplementation with this protein will very quickly activate the immune system, override high levels of nagalase, and enable our own levels of GcMAF to rise. Being an immune modulator, GcMAF can be helpful in every area of health. Reports show that all tumour cancers including breast, prostate, lung, pancreatic and melanoma can be treated successfully. It has been shown to inhibit angiogenesis (stop blood supply to tumours) and revert cancer cells into healthy cells or destroy them. GcMAF has also been shown to reduce the metastatic potential of human cancer cells in culture.

With the ability to modulate the immune system, GcMAF is reported to be effective at eliminating or reducing the effects of nearly all diseases and illnesses, including chronic inflammation and viral infections, autism, chronic kidney disease, depression, acne, colitis, chronic cirrhosis of the liver, crohn's, fibromyalgia, hepatitis, herpes, periodontal disease, ME/CFS, osteoporosis, psoriasis and various types of Immune dysfunction including allergies. Research shows GcMAF can halt deterioration in multiple sclerosis (MS), Parkinson's, dementia and ALS, and due to its ability to modulate the immune system, it can reverse autoimmune conditions such as lupus and arthritis. It is also shown to be helpful with wound healing and increasing energy production at the mitochondrial level.

It is recommended when using GcMAF to be aware of increased sensitivity as the immune system is activated and may attack pathogens and breakdown cancerous areas in the body. When I began supplementing GcMAF and gained good levels of vitamin D from sun exposure, within fifteen minutes I felt a very strong activation of my immune system. Each time I was in the sun I felt mild to strong herx reactions. I also felt the areas of suspected cancer become extremely sensitive.

I found this quite incredible and reassuring to be able to feel my own immune system activating. It gave me huge relief of Lyme symptoms and improvement in areas of suspected cancer. I have used drops and cream successfully. Using moderate strength creams, the herx reactions I experienced were quite mild. Using a newer very high strength cream at times it felt too much for my body to cope. I lessened the amount I was using or at times stopped taking it to give my body time to detox and repair.

Some people with Lyme disease I have spoken to report no herx reaction and immediate relief of symptoms, while others experience severe reactions using just a tiny amount of GcMAF. I have spoken to many people using it for cancer who report very positive results. After reading about how to make your own, I bought some milk kefir grains from a health shop, added milk and colostrum, the colostrum apparently being a vital ingredient which already contains GcMAF. It is recommended to also add specific probiotics, but I thought I would see if it works without them. The results were profound as I felt a very strong activation of my immune system. Homemade GcMAF ingredients:

- Milk kefir grains
- Organic milk (preferably raw)
- Colostrum (preferably organic)

While Kerri Rivera used to recommend GcMAF she now prefers Rerum which she says is more effective with no herxheimer reactions. See below.
ketokerri.com
gcmafproducts.com

Rerum/Chondroitin Sulphate, Oleic acid and Vitamin D
Dr Marco Ruggiero, who worked with Dr Jeffrey Bradstreet on GcMAF, developed what he calls Rerum. Dr Ruggiero thought it was the GcMAF protein in his Bravo probiotic yoghurt that was so beneficial for his patients who had remarkable improvements from many conditions, including cancer, autism, HIV and more. To his surprise when he removed the GcMAF from the yoghurt the health benefits remained. He discovered it was the Chondroitin Sulphate, Oleic acid and Vitamin D combination which he called Rerum which provided the most beneficial results.

I have not used this product but Kerri Rivera has found the autistic children who use the Chondroitin Sulphate, Oleic acid and Vitamin D combination do not have herxheimer reactions in the way they have done when using GcMAF. She has seen incredible improvement in children's overall health, some beginning to speak or regaining speech after many years of being non-verbal.

Medical cannabis
Medical cannabis or marijuana, has been labelled a miracle plant useful in treating virtually all diseases and illnesses including cancer, epilepsy, neurological and autoimmune diseases, anxiety, nausea, insomnia, pain and much more. Cannabis oil is said to be antibacterial, inhibits cancer cell growth, neuro-protective, and promotes bone growth. It also reduces seizures, convulsions, blood sugar levels, inflammation, risk of artery blockage, nausea, vomiting, pain, anxiety, muscle spasms and more.

We all naturally produce cannabinoids. The endocannabinoid system (ECS) is a physiological system with a complex network of receptors playing an important role to bring balance to all biological systems within our body. If our ECS becomes weakened and our own levels of cannabinoids are low, plant cannabinoids which mimic natural endocannabinoids can be very beneficial. Cannabinoid receptors are found in our brain, lungs, liver, kidneys, immune system and virtually all of our tissues, embedded in cell membranes. The medical benefits of cannabis occur when a cannabinoid activates a receptor.

There are a number of different forms of cannabis oil/cannabinoids including CBD, CBDA, CBG, CBGA, CBC, CDCA, THCA, THC and THCV, each containing varying properties which can be more suited to particular illnesses than others. CBD (Cannabidiol), does not contain THC (Tetrahydrocannabinol), the ingredient in cannabis which gives the 'high'. THC is only activated when the plant is heated. A number of specialist say the only time there may be concerns of side effects are when using THC due to its ability to make you 'high' which can cause anxiety.

I have only used a small amount of THC and CBD at different times. I used the THC early in my recovery process and did not like the effect it was having on me. I took one drop of the oil at night time and felt washed out and quite shattered the next morning. I do believe I was probably experiencing a die off effect combined with the effect of the 'high'. Taking the drops at night minimised the effects of the 'high', which I found unbearable on the occasion when I took it during the day. All the same I chose not to continue with it, preferring my other remedies. A year or two later I used CBD oil, which does not give the 'high' and felt immediate and profound benefits, almost as though a switch had been flicked inside me, disabling anything that was affecting my body negatively and activating a strong healing process within.

I am not sure if the CBD simply agreed with my body and the conditions I was using it for rather than the THC, or whether more time on my other treatments enabled my body to be ready for the profound healing effects of medical cannabis. I may never know, but I certainly do know the powerful benefits of this incredible medicine. Due to the amount of research I have seen that pathogens are the underlying cause of most diseases and illnesses, I have a personal belief that medical cannabis also has a disabling effect on these parasites and bacteria allowing the body's own defence systems to regain the upper hand.

While I believe it is important to be careful of overuse due to possible psychosis and paranoia in some cases, as a recreational drug I believe cannabis can be much safer than alcohol. A high quality product with correct levels of the most appropriate oil for certain conditions can be difficult to access, but seems to be more available as many countries take steps towards legalising medical cannabis.

Sommer Healing
My good friend Diane Sommer and I have supported each other sharing all the different remedies and treatments we have tried in our quest for optimal health. Di has shared with me the benefits of many things including NRF2 and has a beautiful skincare product. I highly recommend connecting up with Di.
imunoskincare.com
Sommer Healing (Facebook)

Supplementation
While research has shown our body can create many of the nutrients it needs for optimum immune function, if you are low in some vitamins and minerals it can be a good idea to supplement. Ideally our dietary intake should be sufficient but with the poor-quality soil and growing conditions in many areas this is rarely the case. Particular vitamins and minerals are recommended for protecting yourself against various illnesses. Vit A for measles, Vit C protocols for whooping cough, and with a recent virus outbreak oral liquorice and high levels of Vit C, vit A and Vit D3 have been recommended. See a holistic practitioner.

6 Eliminate Pathogens ... Parasites, Viruses and Bacteria, Mould and Candida

Latest research shows that parasites, viruses and bacteria are one of the main causes of almost all diseases and illnesses. Removing this underlying cause can often result in improvement or recovery from many conditions. Ironically studies also reveal the valuable symbiotic role parasites may play in our body. As mentioned previously, Dr Klinghardt has found that parasites will extract toxins from their host, including heavy metals which otherwise could have been at critically high levels, literally helping them to survive.

That said, once undertaking safe detoxification methods, removal of parasites is one of the most important steps in overcoming chronic illness, as recommended by many practitioners worldwide. Especially for someone who is chronically ill, when killing parasites it can be important to use methods to remove them whole to avoid heavy metals and toxins being released back into the body. Kerri Rivera recommends enemas to do this.

drclark.net   sophiaeducate.com

Breaking down biofilm
Many pathogens create a biofilm, a slimy gel like substance where viruses, parasites and bacteria can live unaffected by our immune system. Many of the drugs and remedies used to kill these pathogens are also unable to penetrate the biofilm in which the nasty little critters hide. Therefore breaking down biofilm is a very important first step in treating pathogens. Many remedies are used to do this, often breaking down the biofilm and killing pathogens at the same time. I have used:

- Essential oils; eucalyptus, cinnamon, peppermint, tea tree, rosemary
- Garlic
- Silvercillin/colloidal silver
- Oxidants; ozone, MMS1/CD, MMS2

Killing pathogens
There are numerous remedies and treatments to kill unhealthy parasites, viruses, and bacteria. Be aware of herxheimer reactions when pathogens are being killed off especially for sensitive people and/or those who have

a chronic illness. I have seen and experienced profound and immediate results using the AmpCoil and Dr Clark's zapper. See the Energy Healing section below for more information. Here are the remedies and treatments I have used to kill pathogens:

- AmpCoil
- Dr Clark's zapper
- MMS1/CD (Kerri Rivera's protocol)
- MMS1 and MMS2 (Jim Humble's protocol)
- Essential oils (organic)
- Herbs
- Redox signalling molecules
- GcMAF
- Homeopathics
- Silvercillin
- Mebendazole, Pyrantel (Kerri Rivera's protocol)
- Ozone

MMS1/CD
Chlorine Dioxide (CD), also called Miracle or Master Mineral Solution (MMS1), is used in a number of protocols. Although there are reports this substance should never be ingested, it has been used for water purification for many years with thousands of people benefiting. To date extensive testing has proven that not one organism is resistant to chlorine dioxide gas. An example of one study - *Inactivation of Human and Simian Rotaviruses by Chlorine Dioxide. Applied and environmental microbiology, May 1990, p. 1363-1366. Yu-Shiaw Chen and James M. Vaughn.*

When you are on death's door and have been sent away by conventional medicine with no answers you ask yourself, 'What else can there be?' A veterinarian whose wife died of Lyme disease suggested I look into MMS1/CD. Since I have been so careful with everything I put into my body I was very reluctant to use this product due to the reports of this substance being chlorine. That was until I researched the science behind it. Bought as sodium chlorite ($NaClO_2$), it has the same chemical composition as salt ($NaCl$), but with one more oxygen molecule. Activated with lemon juice or hydrochloric acid (HCl) it becomes chlorine dioxide (ClO_2). In the body it oxidizes pathogens and heavy metals but does not harm human cells or beneficial bacteria and breaks down to salt and neutralized oxygen. In desperation I gave it a try and had almost immediate relief of many Lyme disease symptoms.

Kerri Rivera's CD protocol *Healing the Symptoms Known As Autism* is by far the most simple yet comprehensive protocol I have followed. As she states it is used to:

- Kill parasites, viruses, bacteria
- Neutralize heavy metals and toxins
- Destroy biofilm
- Reduce or eliminate inflammation
- Stimulate the immune system

Kerri Rivera's online book, *Healing the Symptoms Known as Autism* (second edition), provides detailed step by step instructions which thousands of people around the world have followed for varying diseases and illnesses including cancer, autoimmune and neurological diseases, and Lyme disease. For a number of years I took part in an online support group for people using these methods. I was in discussions with people from all over the world who shared their experiences, the successful improvements, the herxheimer reactions, and the setbacks when something wasn't beneficial. I am fortunate to have had the pleasure of learning about all of the conditions people were overcoming and gaining relief from.

After following Kerri's protocol strictly for a number of years I made adjustments to suit myself. Internationally regarded specialist and Lyme expert Dr Dietrich Klinghardt recommends Kerri's protocol. Senior research scientist Dr Stephani Seneff has discovered that MMS1/CD works to neutralize glyphosate and many toxins in the body. Dr Seneff's research has linked Glyphosate, along with other toxins, to the high occurrence of autism.

Kerri keeps up-to-date with current research and feedback from thousands of people, adding new treatments or remedies as they come to light. Her explanatory book and videos are a must watch. She gives thanks to Jim Humble for building a strong foundation for this work. I found Jim's book, Master Mineral Solution of the 3rd Millennium and later the updated version MMS Health Recovery Guidebook to be valuable resources. This information gave me great confidence that my choice to use this substance was wise. While I found all steps in Kerri's protocol very helpful I chose to do the enemas occasionally rather than daily, but they are recommended and I am sure they are useful for many. Senior research scientist Dr Stephanie Seneff describes the process by which chlorine dioxide destroys glyphosate, breaking it down to useable compounds in the body and discusses the benefits of a maintenance program to protect against toxins.

My recovery using the CD protocol was a long, slow but effective process with mild to strong persistent herx reactions, mild headaches and quite bad brain fog for many months. I persisted, for I knew the bacteria were dying off and I gained relief of all symptoms including muscle cramping, tingling and related anxiety, digestive and neurological problems. Over time my thinking became a lot clearer and my overall health continued to slowly but dramatically improve.

Similar to one of Jim Humble's protocols, *the Perfect Storm Cancer Protocol* uses MMS1/CD mixed with Dimethyl sulfoxide (DMSO), an organic sulphur compound used to draw the MMS1/CD into the cells. I found this to be beneficial and noticed swelling in my breasts which I believe was the mixture working on the cancerous areas.

As MMS1/CD is very strong and can kill large amounts of pathogens in the body very quickly, our body can be overburdened by the die off and too many toxins released, therefore care needs to be taken. It is recommended to strictly follow directions. Some people have not been given safe directions or have rushed into it and had severe reactions. Naturally this puts them off using the MMS1/CD again. I talked to one person with Lyme disease who thought he should use 25 drops instead of one drop because he was very sick. He was horrendously ill with vomiting, diarrhoea and migraine headaches, but recovered fully.

I have spoken to many people who have used Kerri Rivera or Jim Humble's protocols. Despite the usual discomfort of herx reactions, almost everyone who follows these directions carefully and persists with treatment have reported positive results. Some people or companies who seem to have a vested interest in keeping people unwell, put a lot of effort into making this substance look extremely dangerous and criticize the use of it, implying that it is toxic and should never be consumed in any way, despite the fact that it's approved as a water purification agent. I have taken MMS1/CD for six years with no problem. I do not recommend using MMS1/CD apart from water purification as directed. I do recommend learning about it and reading Kerri Rivera and Jim Humble's books. Please seek the advice of a health professional if you have a health concern.

ketokerri.com   genesis2church.ch

MMS2

When I realised I probably had cancer through my back and spine as well as Lyme disease, in a desperate state of extreme illness I chose to use MMS2 as recommended by Jim Humble. When I first found out about this product I was horrified and thought I would never use it. I made the choice not to use conventional poisonous treatments and knew I needed to do something so I did more research into this substance.

I read in Jim Humble's book that what he calls MMS2 is calcium hypochlorite. When dissolved in water it becomes hypochlorous acid (HOCL). Hypochlorous acid is a substance our body makes to kill pathogens and clean up poisons and toxins in our body. As he suggested I searched the internet for scientific information to confirm this. I then chose to go ahead with his protocol. To my surprise MMS2 gave even more relief of Lyme symptoms than MMS1/CD. I also felt it working specifically on troublesome areas of my body including my spine. When needed, it has cleared intense urinary tract and bladder infections within a couple of days. I've also used it effectively on cuts, sea ulcers, and any other infections. At times when I've taken high doses I have felt extremely tired and exhausted, but taking high amounts of probiotics has relieved this. Therefore, I believe the MMS2 probably destroys good bacteria, but I found it well worth using when fighting a serious infection. The fatigue may also have been a die off reaction with the burden of so much disease material breaking down and my body needing time to detoxify and repair. I have been using MMS2 on and off for over four years with no detrimental effects. I have briefly spoken to people using this product who have had good success following directions and there have been no negative reports that I know of. I have used MMS2 successfully for three or four years with no problem. No doubt some sources may be contaminated. I do not recommend taking calcium hypochlorite. I am simply sharing my own experiences. I do recommend learning about it and reading Jim Humble's books. Please seek the advice of a health professional if you have a health concern.

jimhumble.co   genesis2church.ch

Sanitization

Sodium chlorite has been used for sanitization, including in drinking water, food and food preparation surfaces for over one hundred years. **Hypochlorous acid** is used in antiseptic and germicide drugs for wound cleaning, eye drops, baby products, cosmetics and antiseptic sprays. It's

also used for sanitization of hospitals and pool water and since the 1920's has been used in drinking water and praised for saving millions of lives from water borne diseases.
mmsaustralia.com.au   www.miraclemineral.co.nz   genesis2church.ch

Herbal tinctures
There are many herbs which effectively kill the bacteria, viruses, and parasites which cause illness and disease. I have used many herbs a lot which were prescribed specifically for my symptoms. Some herbal tinctures are available over the counter at a herbal dispensary or online, while others may need to be prescribed by a practitioner. There are a number of herbal protocols you can follow for Lyme disease such as the Cowden or Bruhner protocols. Dr Clark's herbal parasite protocol consists of green black walnut hull, wormwood and cloves.
I have also used the liposomal Lyme Cocktail as recommended by Dr Klinghardt which I found to be the most effective herbal remedy. Liposomal, meaning the herbal mixture is put through a process whereby the molecules are encapsulated in lipoids or fats which are absorbed into the body easily. An hour or so before taking the herbal cocktail Dr Klinghardt recommends to take hyaluronic acid which the Lyme spirochetes love to feed on. This lures them out of their hiding places. I found the cocktail to be very powerful. With swelling in both breasts each time I used it early on, I believe it was not only killing Lyme bacteria but also underlying pathogens in the areas of suspected cancer.

Essential oils
Essential oils are beneficial for every aspect of health physically, mentally, emotionally and spiritually. Not only do essential oils fight infections, relieve stress and anxiety and boost the immune system, they also have a frequency which can enhance and strengthen the frequency of our own bodies. I was astounded at the relief ylang ylang gave me, helping my body to settle when I was seriously ill.
Enteric coated peppermint oil capsules provided great relief of severe digestive burning, cramping, tingling and bloating. Peppermint oil down my spine gave enormous relief of severe back problems when I was treating for suspected cancer. Some oils can be applied directly to the skin while others need to be diluted with a carrier oil. Only the highest quality organic essential oils are recommended for ingesting. Some people may be very sensitive to essential oils. I found very little if no herx reaction using the oils.

Oils helpful when addressing bacteria, viruses and parasites:
- Oregano
- Cinnamon
- Thyme
- Tea Tree
- Vetiver
- Lemon
- Lemongrass
- Clove
- Bergamot

Relief of anxiety and stress:
- Lavender
- Rose
- Vetiver
- Ylang Ylang
- Bergamot
- Chamomile
- Frankincense

While addressing suspected cancer:
- Citrus oils
- Clary Sage
- Frankincense
- Lavender
- Lemongrass
- Myrrh
- Peppermint & Spearmint
- Thyme

Ozone

Using an ozone machine I ozonated my water and some olive oil which I ingested. This created a die off with mild to sometimes strong herx reactions. While this method may have been good I was not reaching a level of relief from symptoms that I was hoping for, so it is not on the top of my treatment list. Some people report good success using ozone treatments for Lyme and cancer. There are many people who have had intensive treatment in overseas clinics for Lyme disease. I have spoken to some who report incredible success while others share stories of their condition taking a very bad downhill slide. If you are interested in this form of healing I suggest doing a lot of research and talk to other patients about their experiences.

Homeopathics
I have successfully used homeopathic medicine for myself and my family numerous times for all forms of disease and illness including childhood diseases. Soon after I was bitten by ticks I was given homeopathics. They provided a great deal of relief. Unfortunately, with so many underlying problems I did not know about, symptoms kept returning and I was in need of other remedies and methods. Nonetheless, homeopathics are a very valuable treatement for all diseases and illnesses including reactions to tick bites and the diseases they carry. I have spoken to many people who have used homeopathics successfully for themselves, their families and their pets with no herx reactions reported. Some so-called health professionals believe homeopathics are purely placebo effect. If that is the case, great! It sure works better than other placebos and medication. (See also Homeopathy under Energy Medicine) itchgoes.com.au

Mebendazole/Pyrantel
While it is very rare that I use or recommend pharmaceutical drugs they can be useful and needed at times. Following her work with thousands of children with autism, Kerri Rivera has found it is extremely difficult to rid their bodies of large parasites using only natural products. Therefore she recommends Dr Kalcher's parasite protocol, which uses Mebendazole and Pyrantel. Some parasites killed with these drugs and removed using enemas have been over two feet long. The patients have had huge improvement in their physical and mental health, their aggressive and self-harming behaviours often disappearing.

I know a teenage girl who was having migraines every day. She had pinworm and her mum treated it with over the counter parasite medication. Although they didn't suspect the parasites to be the cause, the migraines disappeared immediately.

Mebendazole and Pyrantel are available from pharmacies.

7 Balance Biochemistry

This from of medicine is without doubt the most beneficial way mainstream doctors can help people to recover from chronic illness. There are increasing numbers of biomedical doctors and nutritionists who use testing methods to determine their patient's levels of nutrients, minerals, genetic inheritance such as MTHFR gene or pyrrole disorder, heavy metals and more. Due to diet, genetic predisposition, pathogens and environmental exposure etc, many people can be lacking or too high in certain nutrients, minerals, hormones and toxins which can lead to serious physical or mental health conditions. Three of my favourite practitioners are Dr William Walsh, Dr Mark Hyman and Trudy Scott ND.

Dr William J Walsh has devoted his life's work to this study. He can look at someone's blood chemistry and determine accurately, which mental health condition they have, be it depression, behavioural disorders such as ADD, ADHD, bipolar, schizophrenia etc. He is then able to help the patient to a strong recovery simply by using individualised natural supplementation. I could write a whole chapter on this but Dr Walsh is the expert and it's all in his book *Nutrient Power*.

Each and every person has a unique biochemistry. Even twins can be very different. One may be high in a mineral or vitamin which the other may be lacking. Therefore, it is very important to undergo testing to make sure you are not making a problem worse by supplementing with something that may be doing harm. For example, high copper leads to low zinc which is directly linked to depression and lowered immune function. Taking a supplement which contains copper will enhance the problem, while supplementing with zinc will reduce copper and bring zinc up to optimum levels, potentially alleviating zinc-related depression. Zinc is also vital for a well-functioning immune system.

There are biomedical practitioners in many countries who will carry out an assessment using laboratory tests of blood, urine and/or hair samples, along with a physical examination, medical and life history data. They will then provide an individualised nutritional supplement program aimed at balancing the patient's body chemistry on the basis of these assessments. Using these methods many people have had great improvement in physical health conditions.

walshinstitute.org   biobalance.org.au
drhyman.com   drnorthrup.com
antianxietyfoodsolution.com

8 Realign Your Body

If our body is out of alignment, it can negatively impact our muscular skeletal system, nervous system and energy meridians, therefore affecting our whole body and every organ within. Many doctors refer patients to chiropractors for help not only with physical pain in the back but discomfort in many areas of the body, migraines, digestive problems, even arthritis and visual problems and much more. Chiropractors do manual adjustments correcting misalignments called subluxations. When the spine is not in alignment the joints can become inflamed and degenerate. The nerves to every area of the body can be impaired impacting every function in our body. Often when the spine is brought back into alignment, with the compression and restriction on the joints and nerves released, the body is able to self-regulate and restore.

I have seen a number of chiropractors during the past thirty years with great benefit. I have no doubt I wouldn't be walking today if not for my chiropractor. My Network chiropractor, operating in the framework of Bio-Geometric Integration (BGI), works to reset the nervous system. He does manipulations of the spine at times when needed, but also works on energy points and meridians in the body to remove blockages. He also assists me using psychosomatic breathing methods to reconnect to areas of my body that I have disconnected from. One day, having asked me to simply breath into and connect with certain points around my body while he made small touches and manipulations of the energy points, he asked me then to wag my tail. I looked at him strangely and wiggled my tail bone. Hearing a click I was amused and quite impressed with his techniques.

Another chiropractor I have seen told me about a particular vertebra in the neck which can cause depression, suicidal and self-harming tendencies if it is out of alignment. By correcting this, he has seen the disappearance of those conditions in some of his patients.

Whether you see a chiropractor, energy healer, osteopath, bowen therapist, physiotherapist, massage therapist or any other form of body worker, doing so to align the body is another vital step toward a full health recovery.

chiropractorbyronbay.com.au
networkchiro.net

9 Exercise

You may think I'm about to tell you to exercise more? No! I am going to warn you about what happens when you exercise while you are chronically ill and the damage that can be done. While exercise is very good for us, if you are in a chronic state of ill-health exercise should be taken carefully. It is good to do gentle exercises to improve blood and lymphatic movement throughout the body such as:
- Walking
- Yoga
- Stretching
- Jumping up and down or bouncing on a mini trampoline
- Tai chi
- Qigong

Our lymph system which has a major influence on our immune system, fat absorption and fluid balance, relies on movement to supply nutrients to the cells and remove waste products, including pathogens, cancerous cells, toxins and debris. Lymph fluid only moves one direction through lymph vessels therefore vertical motion such as bouncing is much more effective than running or walking to move lymph fluid.

But, many people with chronic health conditions often 'crash' for the next few days or week after exercise. This is very common especially for people with Lyme disease and chronic fatigue. This has been linked to mitochondrial dysfunction. I now know it is also related to oxidative stress which is produced by our body's every day functions, including breathing and exercise.

Most people who are suffering from disease or illness have high levels of acidity in their body. When we exercise we build up lactic acid. There are some beliefs that people who are unwell should not do too much exercise to avoid this increase in acidity, which may provide an environment more favourable for pathogens. Also, during the natural process of muscle growth when our muscles have micro tears due to exercise, pathogens have easier accessibility into the muscle fibres.

Each day move your body, do some stretches and a little bouncing on the spot or a trampoline which is great for lymph, maybe a short walk or whatever you feel up to. Try not to push yourself beyond what feels comfortable until you feel confident with your health to do so. Listen to your body.

10 Energy Healing

The term Energy Healing covers a very broad range of therapies which can have powerful beneficial effects on our body, mind and soul. The earth's energy is very healing. Devices and gadgets can be used to access, create or balance energy and protect us from harmful electromagnetic frequencies. Practitioners using many different physical methods such as chiropractic, acupuncture or bowen therapy can assist us to release blockages of energy within our body. Spiritual and emotional healing are also forms of energy healing which I cover in following sections. By removing any blockages of energy or negative interference in our energy field we can enhance our body's own self-healing mechanisms and allow the natural flow of energy and vitality throughout our body.

Protection from Electromagnetic Frequencies / Radiation (EMF/EMR)
The overwhelming amount of EMFs that we are exposed to in our modern age of technology pose serious risks to our health. This is ignored by many companies and health standard regulators who introduce more powerful damaging frequencies into our environment every day via towers, smart meters, baby monitors, alarm systems, phones and devices. At the same time many doctors and scientists around the world are working to find ways to alleviate their negative effects on our health and assist people to recover from the damage caused.
Dr Klinghardt believes EMFs are the number one illness causing factor of our time, even worse than mercury and states that EMFs alter the proteins in our body in the same manner as what happens with nuclear bombs and this damaged DNA can be passed onto our children. He insists that taking preventative measures is a priority when working to overcome chronic illness including Lyme disease.
For a number of years after receiving tick bites I was very sensitive to EMF's which previously did not cause a problem. Many times while sitting inside I could feel the effects of wi-fi. I often yelled out asking my daughters if they'd turned it on and sure enough they had. My whole nervous system was extremely sensitive and I felt a very uncomfortable shaky, humming vibration through my body. Turning the wi-fi off noticeably eased the problem.
There are many mobile phone, personal and home protection devices designed to counter the effects of EMFs such as:

- Tesla Blueshield devices
- K.Dwell chip and stick
- Orgonite (homemade and bought)
- Shielding curtains, blankets, fabrics, wall shielding paint

Dr Klinghardt recommends the K.Dwell chip and stick which help to cancel out negative energy and provide a more healthy frequency pattern. Blushield, as stated on their website is, 'a subtle energy device, mimicking nature but much more powerfully. It stops the body responding to hazardous EMF as its coherent field overrides all ambient EMF fields. The body resonates with the fields from the Blushield device rather than from the many different artificial harmful EMF that now surround us constantly. I felt a noticeable relaxation in my body when using their personal device. I also use the Geocleanse orgone home harmonizer which they state is a healthy, negative charge resonance field generator designed to balance the noxious, unhealthy positive charge resonance created by all forms of EMF/EMR, RF, Wi-Fi, earth radiation and bioplasmic radiation. My sister in law noticed a huge relief when using it. Orgone energy, coined by Austrian scientist, philosopher and psychoanalyst Dr Wilhelm Reich in the first half of the twentieth century, is bio-energy or universal life force energy also known as chi or prana. Orgonite is created by combining resin, classed as organic, and metal shavings, classed as inorganic. Organic materials attract and hold orgone energy while non-organic materials simultaneously attract and repel the energy. Quartz crystal is added to this mixture due to its piezoelectric properties ie when under pressure, such as the constant pressure when resin shrinks, quartz gives off a charge. As a result, negative energy which is constantly attracted and repelled in a 'scrubbing' action is cleansed leaving healthy orgone energy. I wear homemade orgonite pendants which I feel are beneficial.

Earthing
What is Earthing? It is exactly what it sounds like. Connecting with the earth which is a conductor of free electrons. When any part of our skin comes in contact with the earth we absorb large amounts of these negative electrons, whether walking on grass or the bare ground, swimming in the ocean, or hugging a tree. So it is true what they say about hugging a tree but make sure your bare skin is connecting with the tree. The same goes for walking on the earth as synthetic fabrics, soles of

shoes, carpets, vinyl and asphalt all block the earth's electrons from entering our body. I have no doubt being in the ocean and walking on the earth have helped to revitalize my body. Earthing is reported to:

- Reduce chronic disease, Inflammation and pain
- Slow aging
- Calm the nervous system
- Promote deeper sleep
- Lessen hormonal and menstrual symptoms
- Support all organ systems down to the tissues and the cellular function
- Counter the effects of harmful electromagnetic radiation

There are many earthing mats and appliances that can be bought for use when inside the home or work place including a mat to place your feet or any part of your body on, sheets and pillow covers. Specially designed footwear is also available.
donnafisher.net   orgoneffectsaustralia.com.au
earthingoz.com.au   barefoothealing.com.au
klinghardtacademy.com

Energy Healing devices
A lot of past and present research shows that every living and non-living thing, including our own body and any pathogens that may be living within us, has a frequency. In fact, as shown by quantum mechanics, everything in existence is compiled of frequency and sound vibration, sound being the basis for form and shape and that which holds life together. A number of people have devoted their lives to working and experimenting with frequencies including pioneers such as Dr Royal Raymond Rife, Nikola Tesla, Antoine Priore, Dr Bob Beck and Dr Hulda Clark. They have invented and used healing devices with the aim to neutralize negative energies, detect and destroy pathogens which underlie many diseases and illnesses, stimulate bodily tissue to encourage healing and strengthen the immune system, enhance our own healthy energy vibrations and harmonize our body. Some of the devices used for this are:

- AmpCoil
- Dr Clark's Zapper

- Bioresonance
- Rife machine
- Tens machine
- Vega machine
- Theraphi machine
- Scalar wave energy enhancement
- Pulsed electromagnetic field therapy (PEMF)

AmpCoil/Sound Healing
AmpCoil provides our cells, organs and all systems of our body with the optimum frequency they would normally vibrate at. This in turn creates a healing environment, one that is not suitable for pathogens which are often the underlying cause of disease and ongoing inflammation. These harmonious frequencies enable our body's own self-healing mechanisms to work more efficiently.

Developed by a family who struggled for years with Lyme disease, the AmpCoil combines the best of old and new technology. Using biofeedback voice analysis the AmpCoil's tone-generating app BetterGuide can recognize vibrations within our body that are out of balance. A modified Tesla coil projects a fountain-like energy vortex outward creating a pulsed electromagnetic field carrying optimum frequencies which penetrate deeply enough into the body to reach the quantum level of the human cells. This re-tunes and re-shapes the vibrational imbalances found in the body, shifting our core cellular vibration back into balance and neutralizing anything that is foreign to the human body.

AmpCoil has provided one of the most profound healing experiences I have had especially in the areas of my body with suspected cancer. While it is very common for most people to experience rapid results, I was advised this immediate result was most likely enhanced by the good work I had done up to that point. Results show out of one thousand clients five may not respond. This has usually been due to an unresolved problem such as excessive exposure to mould or negative EMR/EMF. During sessions I felt deep and profound changes and improvement in the suspected cancerous areas in my back and spine with enormous relief. Continued treatment showed dramatic improvement in those areas.
ampcoil.com
dianneellis.com.au/ampcoil

Dr Clark's zapper
Dr Clark's zapper sends a gentle electric current of 10 to 500,000 Hz with voltage of 5-10 volts through the body to kill pathogens. Due to scientific advances there is now a computerised version of the zapper which can be programmed to frequencies to specifically counter almost every pathogen and many diseases and illnesses. I found the zapper to be very effective killing a lot of bacteria quickly but, while I was in an extremely sensitive state of chronic illness, it also created a strong herx reaction which was difficult for me to deal with. My daughter had extremely good results with the zapper (see below). I know other people who have used the zapper with excellent results, most of them experiencing a die off reaction before notable improvements.

Learning difficulties, dyslexia, digestive problems, small seizures
My daughter had great results. After just one session on the homemade zapper her digestive problems decreased, energy increased, she no longer had fainting spells and early signs of epilepsy. Her concentration and school work all improved dramatically and her learning difficulties disappeared. A few months later some problems returned but were once again alleviated using the zapper just once. We then used maintenance doses once every couple of weeks until problems no longer returned. Six months after zapping, Lily's school teacher who was providing special learning confirmed sudden improvements in her work. From difficulty with the most simple reading and arithmetic and retaining no information at all, Lily began to excel on all levels.

Bioresonance
With the advancement of technology, computerised bioresonance machines can detect hundreds of frequencies of pathogens, including all sorts of parasites, viruses, bacteria and illnesses. They can even detect emotional conditions, traumas and shock held in the body. Bioresonance can use a person's own energy frequencies to restore the body's ideal energy state. Monitoring the frequencies in our body, it can strengthen and boost healthy frequencies and return them to the body to enhance our wellbeing. Unhealthy frequencies can be inverted or turned upside down and when returned to the body will negate those frequencies in our body. This is said to neutralise or kill many pathogens. I have been amazed at what bioresonance machines have detected in my body, correlating to many of the conditions and feelings that were occurring. I've had treatment with a variety of bioresonance devices over the years

and at times have had profound experiences of enhancement in my wellbeing.

Twenty-five years ago I had a positive experience with treatment from a practitioner using a Tens machine, my health improving dramatically with a lot of energy. Later I had treatment with a German doctor using a Vega machine to treat food allergies and boost my whole system, also with positive results.

Theraphi Plasma Healing
The Theraphi is an electronic device that produces a radiative bio-active plasma field. This super-coherent plasma-wave field restores order to the body's cellular regenerative system, reversing the entropy, or disorder, of the disease process. The Theraphi technology has the ability to provide an influence on general well-being, enhancement of the immune system and reduction of healing times. Some of the benefits and positive results people describe after their Theraphi sessions include: pain and inflammation reduction, higher energy levels, anti-ageing, improved circulation and enhanced immune system responses.

I've had numerous Theraphi sessions with noticeable improvements in my condition. During my first session while sitting in the energy field of the Theraphi, I felt very strong pressure in an area of suspected cancer in my back and chest, which soon eased. Each subsequent session the pressure seemed to move to the next high priority area of concern. It was a strangely positive experience and after each session I felt an easing of symptoms. I have no doubt it had a profound healing effect on a cellular level. I met other people who were also having sessions one being an elderly lady who was in a bad accident when she was young. She had lived with pain most of her life. She experienced relief after one session and complete relief after a few more sessions.

The practitioner I saw is now using the Theraphi in combination with a Tennant Biomodulator, a unique PEMF (pulsed electromagnetic field) therapy device which is reported to enhance the effects of the Theraphi. theraphi.com.au

Protect your own personal energy
Every thought and feeling we have has the potential to deplete our energy if we are not careful or aware of it. Are most of your thoughts negative or positive? Often where we place our thoughts is where our energy goes. People in our lives may be depleting our energy without our realising it. There may even be people from our past who are still plugged

into our own personal energy source. Do you think about a person or event, past or present, and feel bad in any way? If so, your energy is being depleted due to this situation. When we release the emotional charge to this person or event we are able to think about them without feeling upset or depleted. This can be done effectively using many techniques of energy healing and trauma release as listed in the following sections, my favourite being Genome Healing.

How do you feel about yourself? Are you adequate? Are you worthy? Are you equal to other people? If your answer to any of these questions is no, your personal energy is continually being depleted by your own perceptions or the expectations of others. Value yourself. Some of the most valuable people in my life are those who have given me nothing but a smile, a hug, or a phone call, especially when I was seriously unwell.

When we protect and stand strong within our own energy, the more whole and strong we are within ourselves in every way. In turn we are able to participate and give more in every part of our lives. Here are some very simple ways to protect your own personal energy right this moment:

- Be aware of your thoughts and feelings each day especially in times of stress
- Immediately bring the focus of your thoughts back to yourself
- Notice and accept the feelings you have in your body
- Breathe open any areas of tension and allow the energy within you to move
- Detach from negative situations or events
- Look for the positive in life
- Refuse negative thoughts and replace them with positive ones

Energy Healing (Practitioner and Personal Forms)
People all around the world in every culture use energy healing in one form or another. Whether as an individual or with the help of practitioners and shamans, countless techniques can be used to release blocked energy, access higher or more healthy vibrations of energy, engage incredible powers of healing, and balance and enhance the energy systems in and around our body. Some techniques used include:

- Genome Healing
- Breathwork
- PSYCH-K™

- Emotional Freedom Technique/Tapping
- Reconnective Healing
- Reiki
- Kinesiology
- Homeopathy
- Reflexology
- Acupuncture
- Yoga
- Spiritual healing
- Flower and Vibrational Essences
- Crystal Healing
- Colour Therapy
- Shamanic Healing

I have gained benefit from all of these methods at times during the past twenty-five years. Each one can be beneficial to your body, mind and soul. If you tune in to how you are feeling you will be able to work out which technique may be most beneficial for you at this time. Are you feeling emotionally charged or sensitive? If so, Genome Healing and the emotional healing techniques at the top of this list may be most useful. Or are you feeling more unbalanced physically? If so some of the more physical therapies such as reflexology or acupuncture may be suited right now. Listen to your body. Listen to your instincts. You will know what is right for you.

Homeopathy
Homeopathic medicine is made from plant, mineral and animal substances, using a specific process of dilution and succussion or vigorous shaking. The resulting solution is diluted so much that it's difficult to find any of the original particles. Since the medicine cannot act biochemically it is believed to work on the body's subtle energies activating the body's own self-healing mechanisms. There are no side effects or contraindications listed for homeopathic remedies, therefore they are safe for babies, pregnant women, the elderly and people with damaged immune systems.
A homeopath will ask questions about specific symptoms, emotions, thoughts, feelings, body sensations, desires and dislikes to find the appropriate remedy to treat any mental, emotional or physical ailment. Homeopathic remedies are also used to treat deep inner susceptibilities

which founder, Samuel Hahnemann called miasms. These miasms create a predisposition to particular disease states. Therefore, using homeopathy to reverse these predispositions is valuable for everyone, whether healthy or treating a current illness. See your local homeopath or online.
itchgoes.com.au

Kinesiology
Kinesiology is a form of muscle testing to identify imbalances in the body's structural, chemical, mental, emotional and energetic systems. It is an effective way of letting our body do the talking, bypassing all the misinformation and theoretical possibilities we often have swirling around in our head when we feel unwell. When I was seriously ill my practitioner used muscle testing to determine which remedies and foods my body was responding well to. I have no doubt this prevented further deterioration in my condition and enabled a faster recovery. Kinesiology can also be used to determine underlying subconscious thoughts and beliefs which may be having a negative effect on our lives.

11 Emotional Healing ... Release Traumas and The Emotional Connection to Physical Illness

Cancer and many illnesses have been shown to have a direct link to an emotional trauma or event. When we release stress or underlying trauma we're able to heal on a cellular level and restore optimum function. There are many forms of emotional healing, most of these also providing a form of energy healing, including:

- Genome Healing
- Breathwork
- PSYCH-K™
- Counselling
- Psychology
- Neurolinguistic programming

Dr Bruce Lipton has demonstrated how our cells shut down when we are stressed or in a state of defence, the stress hormones affecting our blood chemistry, altering gene expression. Finding areas of our mind, body and soul which have closed down in defence and then reopening them to love is one of the most powerful healing tools we have. This in turn will allow happy hormones to be release into the blood, having a positive effect on blood chemistry and gene expression. While I have found many causes of my ill-health, including toxins and pathogens, for a long time I didn't realise just how much deep tension I held in my body on a cellular level. When a hidden emotional trauma surfaced and I was able to release it, I was astounded at how much tension was released from my body, and in turn how much my body was able to spontaneously heal.

Focus on the positive outcome
We don't need to go delving deep into the past looking for problems. You could be opening a can of worms that is best left alone. Look at what is not working in your life right now such as your health, relationships or work. Make intentions to resolve these issues and focus on the positive outcome you would like to achieve. Whatever is holding you back will surface if and when it is ready to do so. There may be one or more past traumatic events which still hold charge in your body and need to be released. You may also hold hidden negative subconscious thoughts or beliefs which can be transformed into a positive framework. You may

even be carrying ancestral and genetic memory which is impacting your life now. This can be addressed and transformed gently when you are ready to do so.

Due to my life long struggle with ill-health I've spent many years exploring the emotional connection to physical illness. Although it can seem hard to understand, I have no doubt there is always an emotional connection to every illness. Sometimes it's good for us to become aware of what this connection is. Other times just feeling the emotions that come with the experience is all that is needed to move through it.

Are fear and love the same energy?
Many of the pathways within our body with which we feel fear and negative feelings are the same pathways with which we feel love and all associated positive feelings. Think of a time when you may have felt joy or love, but you were in trouble or that love was rejected. That joyful or loving part of you may then have been stifled or shut down. To now access that joyful loving part of yourself, those negative thoughts or feelings may need to be shifted. If we block those feelings of fear, grief, hatred or anger we may also be blocking those pathways in our body which help us to feel happiness, gratitude, love, joy or peace. This tension may cause blockages of energy and blood flow which in turn may cause the development of illness.

If supressed negative feelings arise always remember to allow yourself to feel them, whilst making a conscientious effort towards positive thoughts, intentions and affirmations. In doing so, it is surprising how easily feelings of grief, anger and hurt, can transform into feelings of love, joy and peace. This allows the free movement of energy throughout your body.

Often simple healing processes such as breathwork or Genome Healing will easily enable you to become aware of the underlying emotional connection to physical illness and help you to effortlessly release it. At times, if you are caught in the middle of a chronic illness which seems to have no reason behind it, with no apparent way to regain health, simply being willing and open to becoming aware of the emotional connection or learning may allow you to do so. I cannot emphasise enough how very important this is. Be open to the possibility that emotional healing can happen easily, effortlessly and spontaneously. For a long time it seemed like hard work. It *was* hard work, until I fully surrendered to the process. It is within this surrendering process that true healing can occur with ease.

Negative thought patterns or an awakening?
A pattern of negative thoughts can usually be changed by using awareness and willpower. Trauma or energy blockages held in the body will eventually force themselves out, one way or another, and are usually unaffected, if not strengthened by willpower. This energy will not allow itself to be suppressed. Are you stuck in a rut of negative thought patterns? Or is there a hidden trauma or energy blockage bubbling to the surface ready to be released, and in turn provide an awakening or blissful experience and beautiful way of being?

Retraining neural pathways
If we have been in negative thinking patterns for a long time, the neural pathways in our brain will automatically take us to those negative thoughts, perpetuating the cycle. It can take time and attention to our thoughts to retrain those neural pathways or create new ones. When you catch yourself thinking negative thoughts look for something positive to think about instead. Also be aware if you are drawn into negative thinking by media and the people around you. With repetition, once we have created new neural pathways and patterns of positive thinking it can become an easy habit. PSYCH-K™ is a fantastic tool for this.

Are your thoughts your own?
Some people who are very sensitive can pick up on other people's feelings. Empaths can be so sensitive they take on the feelings and emotions of people around them. This can potentially have a huge impact on their health. If need be, take a step back from people to centre yourself, your energy and your emotions.

Step by step
If all this 'emotional stuff' is new to you it may seem confusing and very difficult to understand what is happening within yourself. Many societies, communities and families do not know how to deal productively with sensitive emotions and differences. If you've grown up with conflict, opening up to sensitive emotions may put you into a state of fight or flight. Recognising this within yourself is important. Some of the methods I describe are very deep and can provide profound shifts within yourself, which at times need to be taken slowly.

Someone to talk to
If you are just starting out with self-discovery, simply having a good listener you can talk to, a trusted friend, family member or acquaintance, can be a valuable first step. Some people might be a bit too close and may not be able to provide a neutral support when emotions are a little raw. Talking with a counsellor, therapist or psychologist can be a huge relief as we release emotions that may have been pent up for years.

Genome Healing

Genome Healing is one of the most incredible forms of mind/body healing I have used. The techniques are revolutionary, simple and extremely effective. Negative feelings can be transformed into a peaceful sense of bliss within minutes. We can directly access and gently release emotions held in every organ and system of our body. This process often reveals patterns in our lives and possibly those which have been carried down through the generations via our genetic and cellular memory. At the moment of conception our first cell is created by the union of the male sperm and the female egg. Genetic cellular memory is carried in every cell as it divides, to eventually create our own unique human body. If there is conflict between this masculine and feminine energy, which could trace back many generations, there may be conflict within our cells, organs, body and our mind.

Allowing your cells, organs and genes to have a voice
Using Genome Healing techniques we are able to talk to our cells and our organs, easily release trauma including genetic and ancestral memory, and return our body to its optimum functioning blueprint. The trauma release method takes minutes and from my experience is permanent. Some other related traumas may arise later and can easily be released. Using powerful quantum mind/body healing techniques we are able to release physical and emotional stress at the cellular level of the body and the subconscious level of the mind. We can literally recreate our reality.
I feel blessed and very grateful to Carol Roberts, the founder of Genome Healing. Since using these techniques I have experienced the most incredible spontaneous transformations in many areas of my life.
genomehealing.com.au
dianneellis.com.au/genomehealing

Breathwork

Breathwork provides an excellent way to reconnect to your inner self, access deep wisdom and love, and reach profound levels of peace and harmony. With awareness on our body and breath, using gentle breathing exercises we are able to unlock and release blocked energy in our body which may have been held from any past traumatic event, birth, or even in the womb. Our body is the home of our subconscious and our spirit. The breath provides a valuable tool for accessing the truth of who we are without the confusion that can happen at times in our minds.

Unlock deep love and bliss from within
Allow the free flow of blissful love and energy throughout your body. Without going into the story of past events, by simply placing our awareness on our breath and body, we can release tension, grief and energy blockages on all levels, physically, emotionally and spiritually. By releasing negative emotions, we are actually releasing blocked energy in our body, allowing it to transform into a positive form of energy and bliss. As we reconnect to deeper loving parts of ourselves which have been shut down, we often feel joy and happiness spontaneously bubbling up from within.

After having my first child I could have been diagnosed with post-natal depression, but I knew I held a lot of grief due to traumatic events in my own childhood which needed to be resolved. My body held huge amounts of tension due to suppressed feelings. Breathwork enabled me to listen to my inner self, to really tune into parts of myself which had shut down due to the loss of two mothers. Those sensitive parts of myself that had shut down were vital to my own ability to be a mother. With guidance I was able to make sense of the feelings I was having in my life, and see they were arising from past events. Developing awareness of where these feelings were coming from cleared a lot of confusion, enabling me to release the negative feelings that had been arising, and connect to some of the deepest feelings of love I had ever experienced.

Breathwork enabled me to experience out of worldly love, bliss and connection and to then ground that into my whole being. This now provides me with an infinite source of love to tap into any moment I choose.

hendricks.com/breathingcoach   jimmorningstar.com
wimhofmethod.com
dianneellis.com.au/breathwork

PSYCH-K™

PSYCH-K™ uses a blend of various tools to change any subconscious thoughts and beliefs which have a limiting and self-sabotaging effect on our lives. Some of these methods which include similar techniques to brain gym and kinesiology are derived from contemporary neuroscience research, as well as ancient mind/body wisdom.

They facilitate change at the subconscious level where at least 95% of our consciousness operates. Weaknesses in the body due to negative subconscious thoughts and beliefs are detected and transformed. PSYCH-K™ is a process that transcends the standard methods of visualization, affirmations, will power, and positive thinking. It is especially effective in the areas of behavioural/habit change, wellness and stress reduction.

psych-k.com
dianneellis.com.au/psych-k

Embody your experiences

Our natural way of being is love, peace, harmony and abundance. If we are not able to live our lives in this way, there is usually somewhere within ourselves that has shut down or closed off. When we unlock trauma and blocked energy we access a very tender and delicate part of ourselves, literally. Many of our emotions are deeply intertwined within our whole being and nervous system on a cellular level.

When practising healing techniques, spontaneous blissful experiences often occur. Occasionally when our energy vibration has changed quite significantly, it can upset the usual equilibrium in our lives. People who are used to us being a certain way may be unsettled with the changes within us, even if they are not consciously aware of it.

At times, the universe will somehow recreate a scenario similar to that which we've been trying to overcome. This is an opportunity to have direct access to the feelings and pathways in our body which have been closed down. Grasp this as a healing opportunity. Feel those areas in your body which have been triggered. They may feel jittery and weak, or tense and tight. Breathe into them. Reassure yourself that all is ok. This time you have an opportunity to become stronger and more resilient, to open up the areas within yourself that have been shut down. This is when true transformation in our lives occurs.

12 Soul Healing

Connecting to a higher love and oneness is very healing for our soul. In doing so we are able to completely free ourselves of any and all of life's worries, if not permanently at least temporarily. There are many ways we can nurture our soul including:

- Connect with nature
- Singing
- Participate in a spiritual practice
- Live your passion
- Meditation
- Gratitude, appreciation and mindfulness
- Shamanic healing
- Genome healing
- Breathwork
- PSYCH-K™

Connect with nature
Take the time to simply watch a beautiful sunrise or sunset, the moon and the stars at night. Sit in nature. Allow yourself to absorb all the relaxing, healing energy of the earth and this universe in which we live. The magnificent, raw and powerful energy of our earth is incredibly healing, invigorating and even euphoric. Use whichever tools are suitable for you to find a deep love and oneness with spirit and universal love.

At times during my life I have experienced many years of feeling alone, unwell and disconnected from society. But something that has always been with me has been a deep connection with nature, and somehow through nature, a connection with spirit. I've spent countless hours just sitting in nature, watching sunrises and sunsets, the animals, birds and the trees, which have provided an incredible sense of oneness. Deep meditation and breathwork has also enabled an almost ecstatic feeling of love within, and oneness with the universe.

Spiritual practice
Whether you believe in a divine creator, God, Krishna, Buddha, or a universal energy, when we connect to a higher infinite and eternal force we have access to the deepest unconditional love. If you feel the desire, prayer is extraordinarily powerful. Use this as a healing tool for yourself

or others. Once you have set your intentions and positive beliefs surrender and trust that life is taking you on a path which is perfect for you. Whether you have a daily routine on your own, Join a spiritual gathering, church or meditation group, when we connect to the pure essence of our soul, spirit and who we are, all that is not that, can melt away.

Live your passion
What are you passionate about in life? What gives you a feeling of oneness or connection, peace, harmony or excitement? Whether it's a sport, singing, gardening, painting, connecting with friends or even your work, finding an activity or practice to fuel your soul gives meaning to life.

Venturing Within ... Going Deeper

Conscious and subconscious thoughts and beliefs
Our conscious and subconscious thoughts and beliefs have an enormous impact on our physical and emotional wellbeing. They also create our reality. Wherever we place our thoughts is where our energy goes. Refocusing our thoughts and emotions towards positive feelings, such as gratitude, caring, love and joy, we can actually bring our heart rhythm, brain rhythms, hormonal, nervous and immune systems into alignment and synchronicity. Every time you have a negative thought or belief about yourself or anything in your life, find the opposite positive thought or belief and affirm that to yourself. Quantum physics shows us that our subconscious thoughts and beliefs not only shape our lives but actually create our reality.

Releasing the trauma of a diagnosis or lack thereof
Receiving a diagnosis can be a huge trauma, especially if it is a life-threatening illness. Simply the word cancer can create enormous amounts of fear. The shock and grief of this type of diagnosis is one of the first traumas to overcome. Many people will only receive very invasive and damaging treatment options. In fear, family and friends will often push the patient to take these options before researching all other available scientifically proven methods. In many holistic and natural circles, the word cancer is not a life sentence, but merely a message to the self that something emotionally, physically and/or spiritually needs to be addressed. Usually all three.

Other times a lack of diagnosis can be extremely traumatic. As myself and hundreds of thousands of people with Lyme disease around the world have experienced, if the testing that is being used is unable to detect what is wrong, being told there is nothing wrong with you when you are seriously ill is a very frightening and traumatic experience.

Along with that often comes lack of support from friends or family when they just don't understand the gravity of your illness and how you are feeling. Acknowledging and releasing this trauma is also very important. While it is good to find your inner strength in these situations it's very important to remind yourself that you do need and deserve medical and personal support. Usually the people close to us are unable to provide the full amount of support we need. This is when online or local support groups can be extremely beneficial.

Make friends with your feelings
During any time in your life when negative feelings arise, particularly persistent painful feelings, try to make friends with them. Often in many societies there is a perception of always being happy and not expressing negative feelings. This can leave us unable to know what to do with those feelings, so we try not to feel or acknowledge them. We try to get rid of them and ignore them, but this can be like trying to dam a river which could potentially burst or become stagnant. Just like a river, if we have stagnant areas of blocked energy this provides a breeding ground for pathogens.

The negative and positive feelings within us are an actual form of energy in our body and need to be allowed to move and transform. If you have any persistent negative feelings that won't seem to shift, just pretend they are your friend. Each time they arise simply think to yourself, 'Oh here is my friend again'. I did this during a very dark time in my life and I was confused when the feelings simply disappeared. I later realised that by training my brain to think of those negative feelings as a positive thing, they were actually transformed to be so.

What is holding you back?
Whether you are wanting to achieve better health, a loving relationship or a better job, if something isn't working out it's usually for one of two reasons. Either the path you are taking isn't right for you and there is a better option, or there may be a subconscious thought, belief or hidden trauma standing in the way of you achieving your goal. If you are unable to achieve something, take the time to feel the frustration around this

issue. Feel where that frustration is in your body. Allow it to its fullest. Allow any answers to come to you. This will often provide the shift that is needed.

Life will provide the healing we need
It has taken me a very long time to realise that every upset or area of disharmony in our lives can be used as a tool for healing. If we set an intention in our lives and something negative seems to occur, it may be a stimulant to reawaken a locked emotion in our body. Use the breathing exercise below to tune in and listen to what is happening on a deeper energetic level. It may be opening up an area within you from which you can fully embrace and experience that which you desire in life.

Finding the Jewel beneath fear
Beneath every negative emotion is fear. Think about it. Every single negative emotion we feel is caused by fear of losing something or someone that makes us feel good or secure. If you have any feelings of fear, whether they are occasional or persistent, explore the depths of those feelings. Feel as deeply as you can how they make your body feel. Often it is here, hidden beneath this fear, where the deepest love within us resides.

Make friends with negative feelings
Sometimes the more we try not to feel hurts or negative feelings within us, the worse they become. And it is exhausting to keep trying to feel good if it's just not working. This is the time to go down into those feelings in your body from an observer's perspective. Welcome those feelings as if they are your friend. Watch them. Notice what happens in your body. This allows energy blockages to move and release.

Rise to the challenge
When something seems too hard, tell yourself, 'I can do this!' Many people with chronic illness feel they just can't keep going. Surrender to the feelings inside, but at the same time look forward to the way you would like life to be and feel. It is during these times that many of us find a deep strength we never realised we had. I have experienced so many hardships and difficulties but now I feel so strong and capable. Challenge yourself. Find your strengths and reward and praise yourself for doing so.

The Power of Positive Intentions and Affirmations

Never underestimate the power of positive intentions and affirmations, especially when we also connect deeply with our breath and our body. You may have done a lot of intention setting and may feel it doesn't work. Keep going with it, just a little each day. Even if you don't notice anything, on a subtle level changes are occurring. Often whatever is holding us back from achieving our intention can surface, making us feel temporarily worse, but this gives us an opportunity to release it and move forward.

When we go to the depths of our emotions, it is from this place within, when we set positive intentions and affirmations, we are able to transform energy and manifest that which we desire. The simple breathwork exercise ahead can be used to tune in to your inner self, your inner wisdom, beyond the constraints of your conscious existence.

While we are using it here to tune in to and release anything holding you back from good health, it can be used for any area of your life that is not working as well as you would like it to. When I first did this exercise I was very unwell. I set the intention, 'I intend to be strong, fit and healthy'. Within two weeks an abscess appeared on my gum. I had been suspicious of a problem tooth for seven years, but I was told it was fine. I had the dead tooth removed and my health improved dramatically soon after. This may be considered coincidence but I have had far too many coincidences to call it just that.

Some positive affirmations for you to practise:
- I love myself
- I am strong
- I am healthy
- I am happy and content
- I am respected in every way
- I am worthy of the best that love and life has to offer

Think of affirmations related to any area of your life that feel appropriate for you and repeat them any time. Make sure the wording is always positive in the present tense as if it is already happening.

Breathwork exercise to release the emotional connection to physical illness

This exercise is best lying down on a mattress. Some soft meditation music can be helpful. For best results put aside one hour or so. Once you are very familiar with the process it can be done within minutes during your daily life.

1. To start with set positive belief statements for yourself such as:
   'I am strong, healthy and well'.
   'I am safe'.
   This will activate a self-healing process within your body even if you don't notice it.

2. Set intentions/positive belief statements about anything you would like to achieve in your life:
   'I walk or run each day'.
   'I have a great job that I love'
   'I have a wonderful relationship'.
   'I am understood'.

3. Close your eyes. Think about the condition or illness you are concerned about. Feel how it feels in your body. Is there a thought that comes to your mind? Is this relevant to your condition? Still with your eyes closed, focusing on the area of concern, ask yourself some questions such as, 'What is the underlying cause of this illness?' 'What am I needing at this time?' Ask any questions that you feel appropriate. Allow an answer to come to you or maybe visualise an empty blackboard and watch an answer being written on it. You may or may not become aware of an answer or something may come to your awareness at another time. Either way is fine.

4. Again with your eyes closed, focus on the area of concern in your body. Breathe nice full relaxed breaths into the area. Feel the area. Notice any sensations in your body such as hot, cold, tingling, cramping. Allow the feelings to move, change or stay the same, to strengthen or weaken. Just observe them. You may not be aware of any feelings. If so, notice the feeling of nothingness. Images, memories, pictures or colours may come to your mind. If so, there is no need to do anything with them. Just notice them and bring your awareness back to your body and your breath. Be aware of any emotions that arise. Again, just notice them and always bring your awareness back to your body and your breath.

5   Allow any feelings within your body. Do not go looking for negative emotions or go into the story of any past events. If there are hidden feelings of grief, sadness, guilt, or sorrow etc that need to be released, they will do so spontaneously. Just feel the feelings that arise and allow them to their fullest, always bringing your awareness back to your body, your breath, and the present moment.

6   Be open to the possibility of only positive emotions and feelings arising. Focus on how they feel within your body and allow them to amplify.

7   State your positive affirmations and breathe those beliefs into every cell of your body, particularly into any areas where there was tension or negative feelings. Visualise the outcome you would like to achieve. Feel those feelings, breathing them into every cell of your body.

8   Be aware of any thoughts of inspiration or insight that come to you. Write them down if you wish. If you have any visions you may like to draw them. Some coloured pencils may come in handy.

By simply bringing your awareness, energy and positive affirmations to the area of concern you will activate a healing process. This may take practise or you might have feelings of relief, happiness, joy or a deeper feeling of oneness and peace.

Daily breathing exercise
The principles of the breathwork exercise above can be carried out in your everyday life. As you go about your day, remember to notice how your body feels. Allow the feelings in your body. Notice any areas of tension or stress. Don't fight them. Just allow them. Breathe into them. Relax. It might take practise, but this can all be done no matter what you are doing in your day, even when you work and while talking to someone. This simple yet powerful process allows the free flow of energy in your body. It also helps you to be aware of and protect your own personal energy.

Daily emotional awareness exercise
Each day keep a close vigil on your thoughts. Are you thinking positive life enhancing thoughts? Or are your thoughts negative and disheartening? Remember that every thought we have releases hormones into our blood stream, affecting every function of our body. Training and refocusing your thoughts to be positive, while still allowing your true feelings, your true self within, is the key. There may be times of stress and difficulty, or negative emotions from past events that we need to work our way through. Allow yourself to do so, accepting and acknowledging the full depth of those feelings. Then bring yourself back to a positive mind set. When you notice any negative thoughts creep in, stop them. Once again, find the opposite positive thought or belief, and reaffirm that to yourself. In doing so you are actually changing the neural pathways in your brain, and this way of positive thinking will become a habit.

Each day practise repeating positive affirmations about yourself and your life as if it is already happening. Remember to always use positive wording in the present tense such as, 'I am strong', 'I am healthy', 'I have a loving relationship with my partner, children, friends or workmates', 'I am successful.' Even if things in your life are not yet happening as you would like them to be, even if you don't really believe it will happen, by doing this exercise you are changing your subconscious beliefs which will create a positive change.

Determination and commitment
Whatever may be causing disharmony in your life, whether a health condition, something from the past or in your day to day life, we often need grit, determination and commitment to ourselves. As a society we have lost sight of the sensitivities and strengths within us, the connection with spirit and soul. Our outer world, friends, colleagues, the media and internet can very easily distract and confuse us to what is most important for our spontaneous joy and happiness within. Commit to yourself and make changes that feel right for you, honouring and respecting your true self.

> *'Beneath all negative feelings, profound feelings of love, joy and peace can be discovered. Sometimes, the most precious jewels are found within the depths of darkness. Shine a light on the darkness and it disappears. The joy and beauty within are truly blissful'*

Venturing Out ... With Your Inner Self

In an ideal world each of us would feel safe to allow the deepest most sensitive parts of ourselves to be seen in every area of our lives. But living in this physical reality, that is not always appropriate or possible. When we become in touch with these sides to ourselves we need to feel safe and supported to live from that place of sensitivity. At times we need to make changes to our outer world so our inner self can thrive.

Letting go of that which no longer serves you
Particularly during times of illness and hardship, we find our lives changing. We find ourselves changing. Some people are able to be there for us during these times of difficulty. Some people in our lives may no longer understand us and the whole dynamic of our relationship changes. Often while we are unwell we become needier, and some people who we hope will be there for us are not able to meet those needs. Often we are not able to meet the needs of others in the way we have previously done, which can upset them. It can be very traumatic for all parties involved.

Some people deplete our energy and it is best to let those people slip away out of our lives, or make sure you protect your own personal energy. It might upset people when you prevent them from tapping into your energy but it is vital for your own health and wellbeing. I have learnt that when we let go and trust, the people who are meant to be in our lives will be. Letting go of people can be painful, but it is always better for both parties. You may need to let go of someone you love, but you don't need to let go of that love. That is your own feeling to hold onto if you wish. Things may change and bring the person back into your life at a later time, or your lives may go separate paths.

It is also important to let go of any situations or activities that are no longer serving you. Don't do something because you feel you should or you are obliged to. Make sure you are doing what makes you happy and uplifts you. If it isn't doing so, it may be time to let it go and find more rewarding activities in your life. Allow changes to unravel as they are meant to, easily and effortlessly. Let life unravel easily and effortlessly.

Hold on to what is important to you
While it is essential to let go of what is not serving us, it is vital that we hold on dearly to those we love and that which is important to us. What in your life feeds your soul, nourishes and nurtures you and makes you feel good just thinking about doing it? Who are the people that support

and uplift you, care for you and make you feel loved and cherished? Who in your life doesn't care if your hair is brushed or whether you are happy or sad, can sit beside you in your darkest moments or soar alongside you when you are flying high? Who do you feel safe to be around when you expose the most sensitive sides of yourself. These are the people and the things that give our lives true meaning and purpose.

Healing Relationships
If you are having difficulty, or you are unhappy with a relationship in your life, step back for a moment and consider what might be happening on an energetic level. Temporarily put aside what you are seeing or hearing. How are you *feeling* about this relationship? How are you feeling about the other person and within yourself? Rather than trying to change the circumstances around this relationship, go within yourself. Feel the feelings this disharmony has created, the energy blockages within your own body. There is no excuse for another person's bad behaviour, but it can at times bring your awareness to an area of yourself that has been shut down, triggering you to go within and find a deeper love within yourself.
Feel where the tension or angst is in your body. Breathe nice full relaxed breaths into those areas stretching them open, breathing life into those areas of tension. Like an observer, watch the feelings. Allow them to move, shift, strengthen or weaken. Feel them to their deepest depths, while watching and observing with curiosity to see what they might do.
Be open and aware of where these feelings may have originated and allow any other related feelings to arise. If this does happen allow it fully, but do not go further into the story of these events. Simply acknowledge where these feelings came from and allow them to their fullest. If you're not aware of their origin simply acknowledge and feel them.
Now set positive belief statements to override any trauma held within you from these events or feelings, eg, 'I am worthy', 'I am understood', 'I am loved', 'I am safe'. By doing this practice you may realise how some feelings that you hold within yourself are reflected in the people around you and maybe have done so for much of your life. Some of these feelings may even be a genetic memory carried down through the generations, which will be much better to be cleared from your psyche. This can be done very effectively using Genome Healing methods.
There are times when we need to address conflicts or differences with another person. There may even be times when we need to let go of people or relationships. But always be open to finding any areas of

yourself that may have shut down in defence due to past hurts and look for ways that you can love yourself more. This self-loving vibration will in turn attract more love into your life and can facilitate spontaneous healing of self and relationships with those we love.

Emotional responsibility
Taking responsibility for our own feelings and emotions is very empowering and vital for healthy relationships. It is important to be aware of the effect of our own words, body language, thoughts and feelings towards others.
Letting go of feeling responsible for other people's feelings is also crucial. Although we may try, at times we might not be able to meet the expectations of those around us and vice versa. This can lead to underlying feelings of guilt or resentment. One of the most profound shifts happened in my life when I stated that I am not responsible for my mother's feelings. Without realising it, somewhere deep within, I'd held feelings of being responsible for the distress that was created when my mother fell pregnant with me as a teenager. No matter what the circumstances were, this was a belief I had taken on which was having a huge effect on my mental, emotional and physical wellbeing. Taking care for, but not feeling responsible for another person's feelings is important for our overall mental, emotional and physical wellbeing.

Accept yourself and others
It's the quirks and eccentricities in life that add colour and flavour to our world. Have you ever been told you're too quiet, too loud, too outrageous, too dull? Maybe too smart, too dumb, too controlling or not assertive enough? Some people may have more emotional intelligence than mathematical genius. Some are leaders while others are happy to work quietly in the background. Claim your strengths and love them! Love yourself and allow others to do the same.

Stay strong in your convictions
It is always good to be open to different points of view and different ways of life. What you believe is right or wrong may simply be a different perspective held by you and other people. This may change many times during your lifetime. Every person's reality in life is different. However, the essence of who you are, what is important to you, your thoughts, feelings and beliefs about yourself and what you value in life, do actually create your reality and your sense of self. Always hold on to that.

Love; the linchpin of life

Love is at the core of all life and everything we do. If life isn't quite working or feels too difficult at times, always come back to the love within. The love of trusted friends, family, pets or nature. A solid love that is unshakeable. Divine or universal love. This will ground you and give you security. So many distractions, motivations and fears in life can take us away from true love. Check in with yourself often to see if you're operating from a place of genuine love. Or have fears and desires distracted you? Difficulties can often push us to find a place in ourselves we have shut off. Be brave. Sit within any intense feelings you have, allowing them to show you a deeper more content love from within. When we live from this place of heart centred love in every area of our lives, the richness and contentment we feel is profound.

Gratitude, appreciation and mindfulness

Appreciating and being grateful for what you in your life in each present moment is one of the most effective ways to feel happy. No matter what situation you are in or how difficult life may get, we can look for the pleasure in the simple things in life and be grateful for them. Our friends and family, a walk in the park, watching a sunrise, eating a simple healthy meal, lying in a warm soft bed. The beauty of a flower, the warmth of the sun. A car to take us where we need to go and a car jack to change a flat tyre. Rather than being upset with a flat tyre, imagine how irritating it would be if you didn't have a spare! Even just to be able to take a nice full relaxed breath. For an asthmatic this is bliss. The more we can find in each day to be grateful for, the more we will notice what we have in our lives to be grateful for. This feeling of gratitude will also release feel good hormones into our body and have a positive effect on every cell and all the systems of our body.

Give yourself permission to feel good

Many of us, on a conscious and/or subconscious level, hold negative belief systems carried down from our ancestors, such as 'Life is hard', 'I don't deserve', 'If someone is too nice they must want something'. Give yourself permission to feel and fully embrace the joys of life. Find the opposite of those negative thoughts and beliefs and repeat them to yourself, eg 'Life is easy', 'I deserve the best', 'People are generous'.
Ask yourself, 'How good can I feel? How much love can I allow into my life?' What makes me truly happy? Follow what really makes your heart sing.

My Ongoing Health Recovery Protocol

I am deeply relieved and grateful to say I've had enormous success repairing my body and my immune system. If we eat well and all of our systems are functioning properly, unaffected by pathogens or toxins, we are generally able to gain all the nutrients that are needed for our body's optimal function. The miracle of our body is that it can produce everything it needs to repair itself unless something has thrown its usual processes out of balance.

Due to the extent and length of the chronic health conditions I've experienced, I continue working to ensure I clear all remnants of disease and anything which is not nurturing to optimum health. After years of desperately working out what I can take each day just to make it to the next, now I only take a couple of remedies or immune activators if I feel the need or if I've been exercising a lot. With thanks I will happily consult a naturopath, homeopath, holistic or mainstream doctor, or any other practitioner if need be any time in the future.

My protocol now includes:
- Daily kidney and liver cleansing herbal teas
- Bicarb or hydrogen water (either taken internally or on the skin)
- Diatomaceous earth, bentonite clay and/or chlorella
- Fermented food and drinks
- MMS1/CD
- NRF2 and redox signalling molecules every day to continue strengthening my own immune function and self-healing mechanisms
- AmpCoil
- Regular chiropractic, massage etc
- Essential oils
- For acute situations I may follow Jim Humble's MMS2 instructions (this is not a recommendation)
- Herbs if and when needed

Every day I look for happiness and contentment with the simple things in my life, grateful for each one. I regularly practise the breathing and emotional release exercises above depending on what is happening in my life. Having released the energy blockages and grief from numerous big traumatic events in my life there are now, at times, little upsets or traumas that come to my awareness which I usually release in minutes. Occasionally there are bigger issues which take a longer process of unravelling. Each time I do so, I'm taken deeper to the true essence of myself, untainted by the constraints and superficial restrictions of the material world. A deeper more peaceful, loving and happy place within myself. In turn, I feel my whole body and every system within relaxing, calming, energising, and igniting a passion for living a wholesome, healthy and vibrant life on this earth.

I wish you well on your journey to optimal health, wellbeing and happiness. If you or a loved one are ill or have even been given a terminal or permanent diagnosis, always know that miracles can and do happen every day. Be open to learning. Remember to listen to that voice within, your own inner wisdom, and allow yourself to be guided by it. Most of all, find the courage and allow yourself to let go of anything within you that is dampening your spirit, your love for life and love for yourself. Allow that love within to melt away any resistance to living with optimum health and happiness. The power to manifest a beautiful life of love and contentment is within each of us.

Connect with Di

dianneellis.com.au
Facebook – Di Ellis Health and Photography
Instagram – di.ellis

A special thank you Maggie Hamilton
Writing and publishing this book has been an
incredibly healing process. Your beautiful kindness,
generosity and nurturing has supported me all
the way. Thank you for helping me to arrive
at my special place.

Di Ellis

www.ingramcontent.com/pod-product-compliance
Lightning Source LLC
Chambersburg PA
CBHW032031290426
44110CB00012B/750